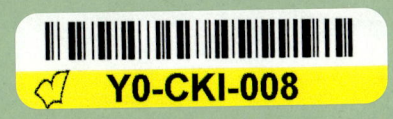

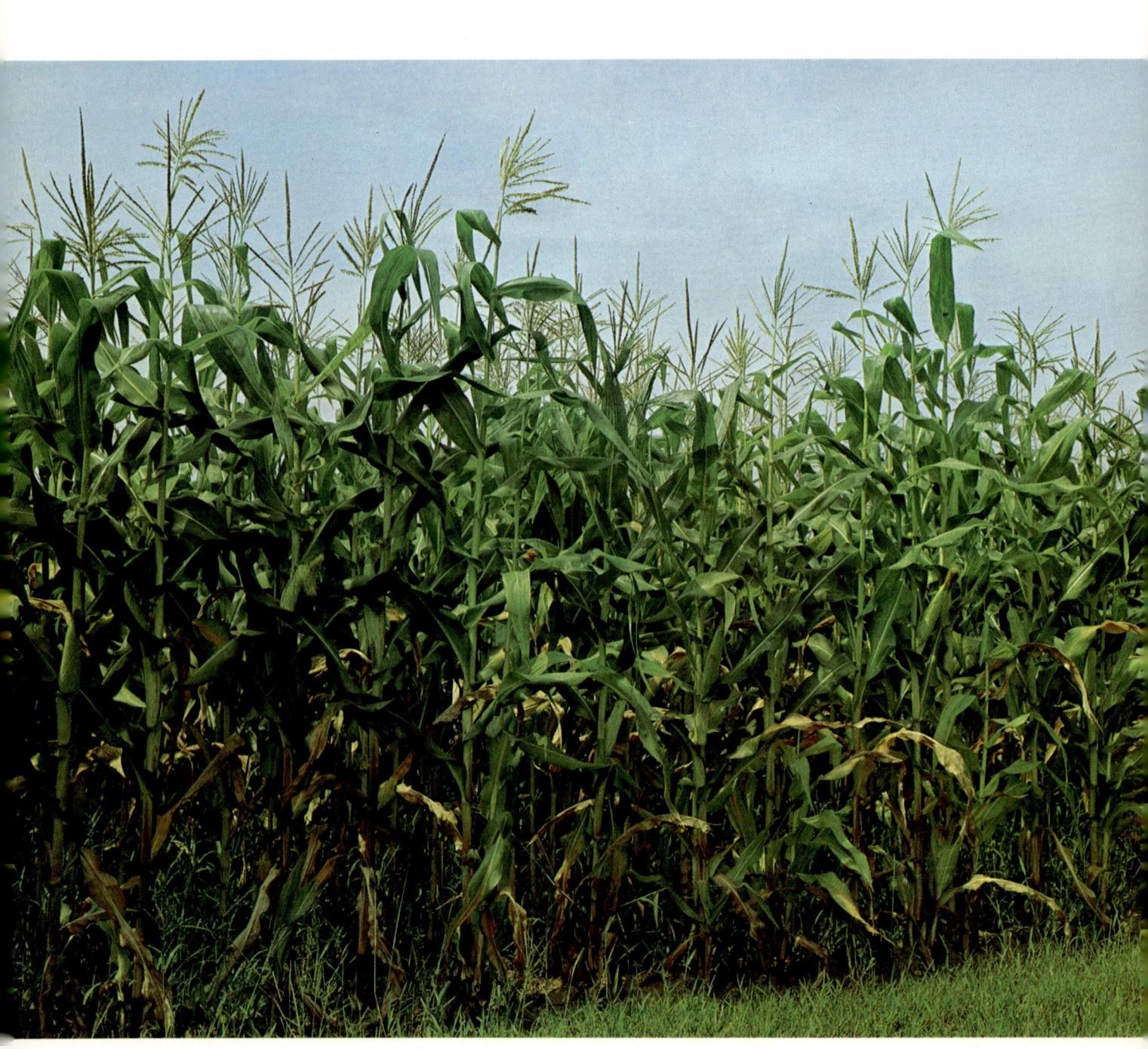

SCOPE® MANUAL ON NUTRITION

MICHAEL C. LATHAM, M.D.
ROBERT B. McGANDY, M.D.
MARY B. McCANN, M.D.
FREDRICK J. STARE, M.D.

The Department of Nutrition
School of Public Health
Harvard University

PUBLISHED BY THE UPJOHN COMPANY, KALAMAZOO, MICHIGAN

Baird A. Thomas
Editor

LIBRARY OF CONGRESS CARD NUMBER 71-112745

© 1970, THE UPJOHN COMPANY, KALAMAZOO, MICHIGAN.
NO PART OF THIS WORK MAY BE REPRODUCED OR UTILIZED IN ANY FORM OR BY ANY MEANS, ELECTRONIC OR MECHANICAL, INCLUDING PHOTOCOPYING, RECORDING, OR BY ANY INFORMATION STORAGE AND RETRIEVAL SYSTEM, WITHOUT PERMISSION IN WRITING FROM THE PUBLISHER.

THE UPJOHN COMPANY, KALAMAZOO, MICHIGAN S-9232

Table of Contents

Preface 7
Introduction 8
Recommended Dietary Allowances of Nutrients . . 13
Special Medical Problems With a Nutritional Component
    Nutritional Concepts in Heart Disease 16
    Obesity 19
    Dental Caries 22
    Osteoporosis 26
    Iron Deficiency Anemia 27
    Protein-Calorie Malnutrition of Young Children . . . 28
    Xerophthalmia-Keratomalacia 37
    Thiamine Deficiency Syndromes Including Beriberi
        and the Wernicke-Korsakoff Syndrome 38
    Pellagra 41
    Scurvy 43
    Rickets and Osteomalacia 44
    Endemic Goiter 48
Nutrients
    Protein 53
    Carbohydrate 54
    Fats 54
    Water 56
    Minerals 56
    Iron 56
    Calcium and Phosphorous 58
    Iodine 60
    Fluoride 61
    Sodium and Potassium 63
    Magnesium 64
    Copper 65
    Sulphur 65
    Trace Elements 65

Vitamins
    Vitamin A 66
    Thiamine (Vitamin B$_1$) 67
    Riboflavin 68
    Niacin (Nicotinic Acid) 72
    Vitamin B$_6$ 74
    Pantothenic Acid 76
    Cyanocobalamin (B$_{12}$) 77
    Folacin 79
    Vitamin C (Ascorbic Acid) 80
    Vitamin D 83
    Vitamin E 86
    Vitamin K 88
    Biotin 89
Finale 91
Appendices
    A. Table of Sodium, Potassium and Magnesium Content of Selected Foods
    B. Table of Food Values
    C. Approximate Cholesterol Content of Selected Foods
    D. Table of Desirable Weights for Men and Women Aged 25 and Over
Acknowledgements

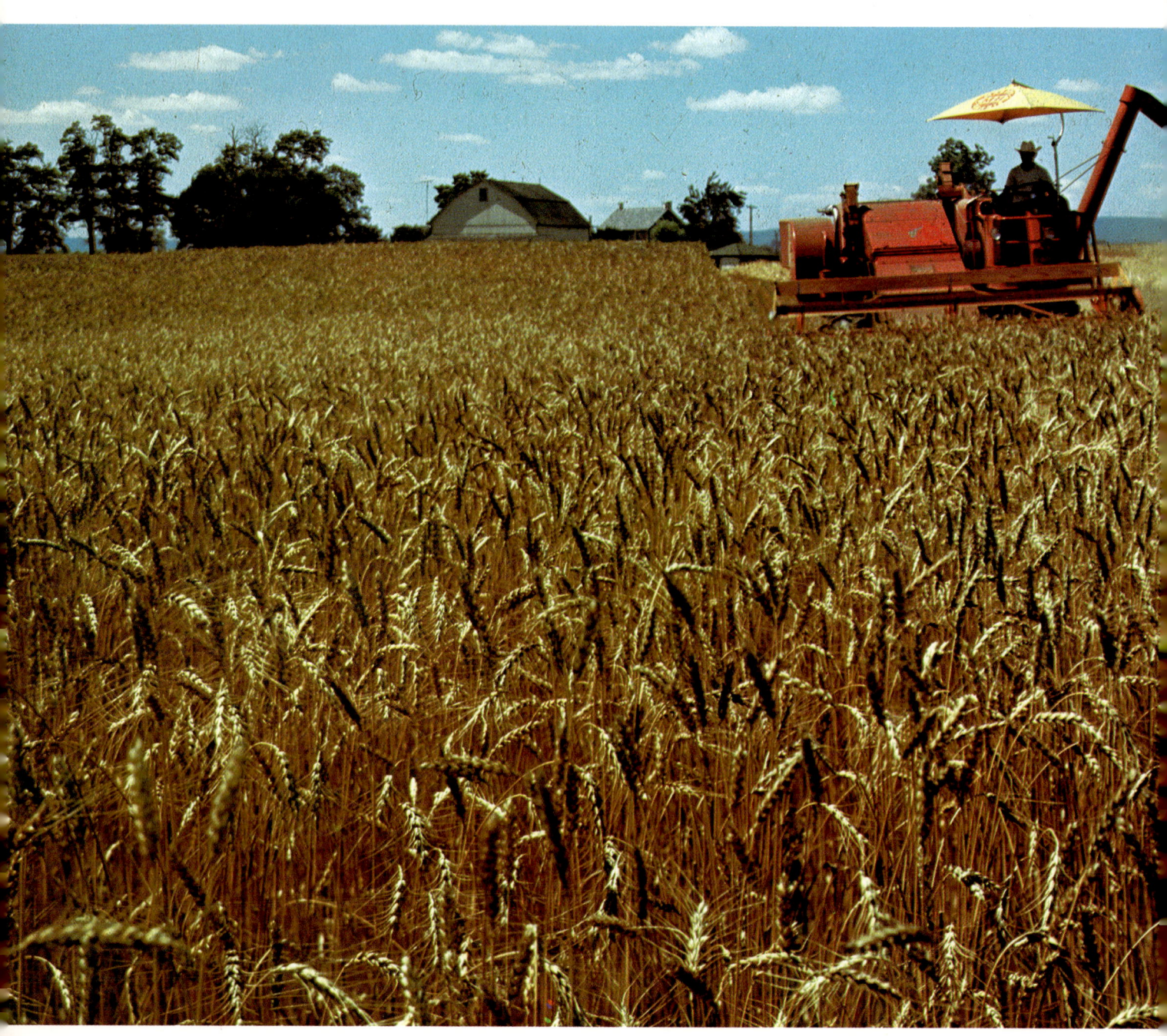

Preface

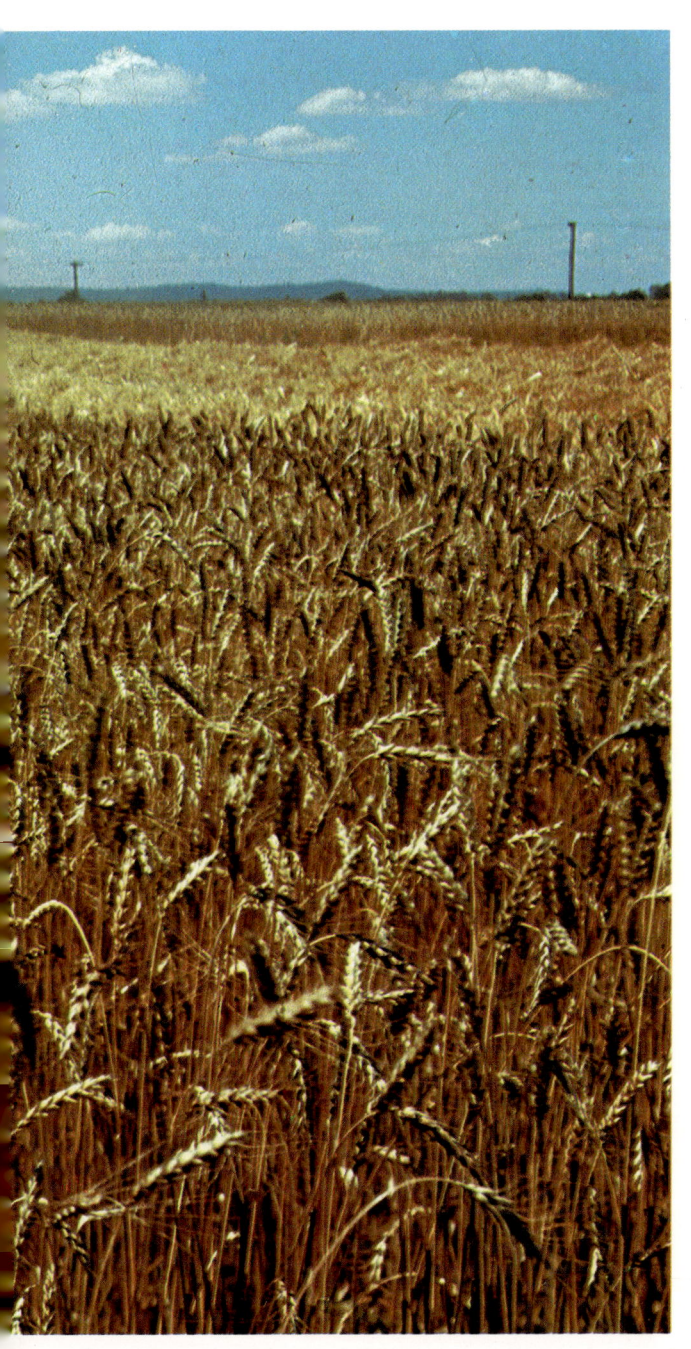

Our major job has been, and is, teaching, training, researching, and sending "our products" elsewhere to teach, train, research, and be of service in nutrition, which we consider an important and a largely neglected field of health and medicine. When the idea, and then the first draft of this Manual of Nutrition was born, my three collaborators were all young physician-nutritionists, members of Harvard's Department of Nutrition. But before this Manual was completed, two of my associates had left us. Dr. Michael Latham is now Professor of International Nutrition at Cornell University in Ithaca, New York, and Dr. Mary B. McCann is with the United States Public Health Service in a position of key responsibility relative to the nutrition surveys being conducted in many of our states. I am indebted to both of them for their help, particularly Dr. Latham who has continued to do more than his share.

Dr. Robert B. McGandy, an Associate Professor of Nutrition at Harvard, has played an important role in the preparation of the final drafts of this Manual. I am most indebted to him. In addition, other members of Harvard's Department of Nutrition–Drs. D. M. Hegsted, J. Mayer, S. Gershoff, D. S. Bernstein, R. and Mrs. J. Hattner have had a hand in either writing or reading various sections of this Manual.

We all hope that this Manual, which is not a textbook, not a reference book, but a manual on nutrition primarily for medical students, house officers, and general practitioners, will teach a little nutrition and stimulate considerable interest in learning more nutrition and its application to problems of contemporary medicine and health.

Fredrick J. Stare, M.D.
Professor of Nutrition
Chairman, Department of Nutrition

Introduction

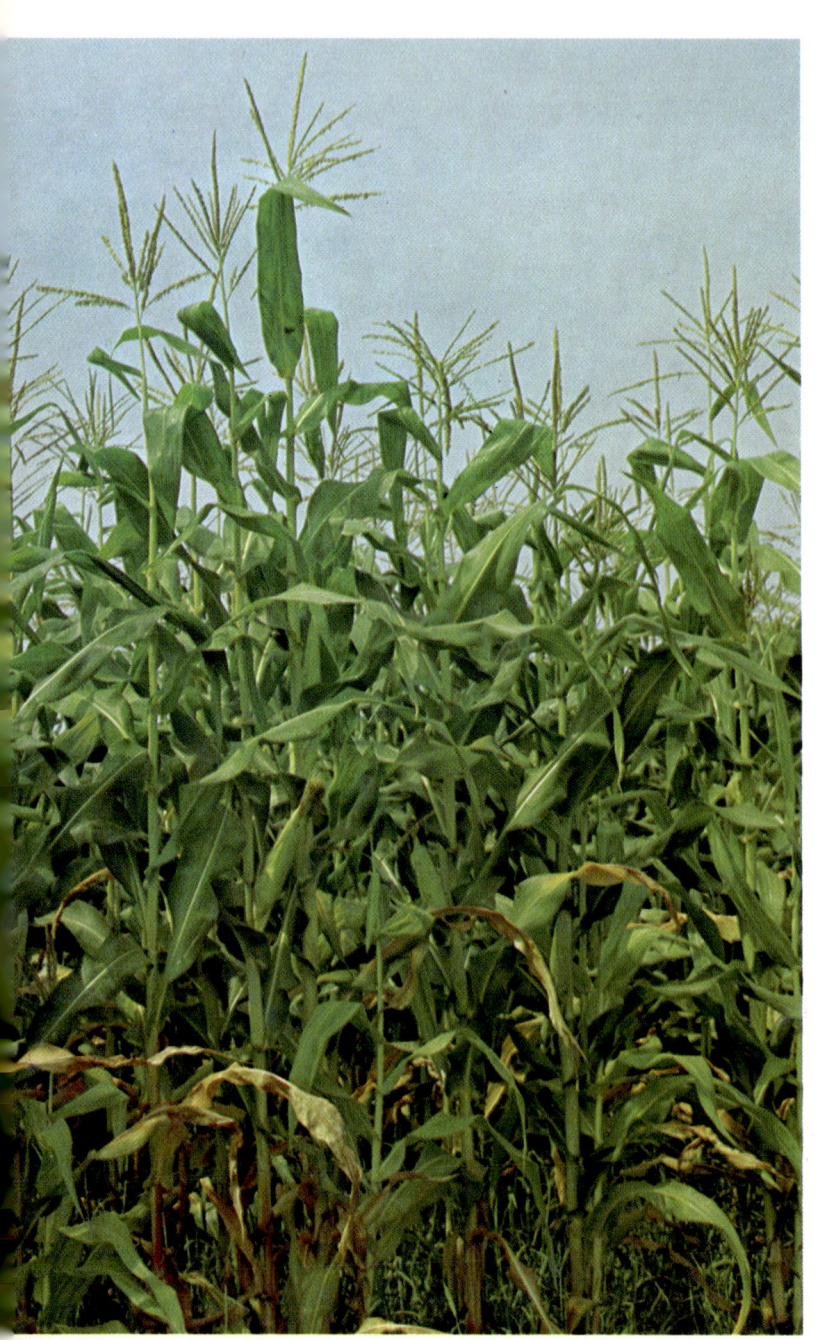

Nutrition is an important factor in the etiology and management of several of the major causes of death and disability in our contemporary society. Arthero-sclerotic vascular disease, obesity, tooth decay, osteoporosis, and diabetes are common diseases in this country in which nutrition is closely involved.

In the developing areas of the world, malnutrition of early childhood due to protein-calorie deficiencies as well as a host of infectious diseases made worse by poor nutrition, iodine deficiency goiter and blindness due to lack of vitamin A are a few major health problems directly related to inadequate nutrition.

Iron deficiency anemia and dental caries are widespread problems of inadequate nutrition which have neither geographic nor socio-economic boundaries. Even in highly developed societies, there may be large segments of the population in which hunger and undernutrition impair physical and mental performance.

As yet, instruction in the principles and practice of proper nutrition remains almost nonexistent in most of our medical, dental, public health and nursing schools today. The biochemical and physiological basis of nutrition is frequently no longer a part of the pre-clinical sciences. Clinically the major emphasis has been placed more on drugs and surgery than on the nutritional aspects of management and almost no attention is paid to the role of nutrition in the prevention of illness.

What is nutrition?

Nutrition is the science of food, the materials or nutrients in food, what they do and how they interact—all in relation to health. Nutrition comes from food, good food that one enjoys (for eating has always been one of the pleasures of life); from food in variety so that it supplies all of the 50-some known nutrients that are necessary for proper nutrition so as to provide the best of health that one's genetic or hereditary background permits.

Variety in foods consumed is the keystone to proper nutrition because no single food provides all the known nutrients, not even mothers' milk. Consuming no more calories than required to reach and maintain a desirable body weight is also important. This depends in large part on one's physical activities because muscular activities are the only way one has of using up calories beyond those needed for basal metabolism, doing your job and whatever you do with leisure or spare time.

In the last decade or so, as will be pointed out later in this manual, it has been found that the type of fat in the diet, as well as the cholesterol content of the diet and the caloric balance are important factors affecting the level of cholesterol in the blood. The latter is one of the factors, and a most important one, in affecting susceptibility to coronary heart disease and cerebral hemorrhage. The higher the level of cholesterol (and also other fats) in the blood, the greater the chances of developing these common causes of death, particularly when it is in association with other conditions such as an elevated blood pressure, family history of death before life expectancy, diabetes, cigarette smoking, overweight, lethargy or infrequent physical activity.

Nutrition as a science can be divided into six main categories–protein, carbohydrate, fat, minerals, vitamins and water. The first three categories are the only ones that provide calories; that is, protein, carbohydrate and fat. Four calories per gram are provided by both protein and carbohydrate. Fat provides slightly more than twice as much, 9 calories per gram.

Alcohol is not considered a foodstuff but from time immemorial it has been consumed by man in various fermented and distilled beverages and it does supply about 7 calories per gram so it must be considered in evaluating one's total caloric intake.

Minerals and vitamins provide no calories but function in the many metabolic processes whereby one obtains and utilizes calories from foods, builds and then maintains body tissues. Minerals also function as vital constituents of many body tissues such as the iron of hemoglobin, myogloblin, and the cytochromes and the calcium and fluoride of sound teeth and bones.

Water, in addition to making up some 70% of the total body, is essential for the absorption of many nutrients, the elimination of body wastes via the urine and feces, and the maintenance of a normal body temperature via evaporation of water from the lungs and skin. While water provides no calories or vitamins it may provide calcium and magnesium in the case of "hard" waters and when fluoridated, either naturally or artificially, is the only important source of the mineral nutrient fluoride. This mineral nutrient is not only the single most important factor in lessening tooth decay (by 60-70%) but is important in lessening the incidence of osteoporosis in ageing and it may be important in lessening the incidence and severity of soft tissue calcification as for example in hardening of the arteries.

Nutrition is important in modern health and medicine–in improving and maintaining good health and in improving poor health. It is hoped that this manual will stimulate students of the health professions—medicine, dental, public health and nursing—as well as practitioners of the health professions, to learn more about nutrition and apply it for the benefit of mankind.

How prevalent is malnutrition in the USA?

This depends in part on what we mean by malnutrition. If we mean illness or poor health resulting in part from poor nutrition, it is widespread and among all economic classes. For here we would include tooth decay due to inadequate intake of the mineral nutrient, fluoride, and tooth decay is almost universal. We would include osteoporosis contributed to by lack of fluoride and this is radiologically demonstrable in 50% of adults over sixty years of age.

Related in part to malnutrition is atherosclerosis as manifested by coronary heart disease, cerebral, renal and peripheral artery disease. Essential hypertension can be lessened by decreasing the intake of the mineral nutrient sodium, and may possibly be caused by too much sodium and aggravated by obesity. These cardiovascular diseases are responsible for well over half the deaths in this country. Iron deficiency anemia is certainly prevalent in all societies.

The acute and severe vitamin deficiencies as manifested by the classical nutritional diseases—scurvy, pellagra, beriberi and xerophthalmia—are not common in the USA, but they are prevalent in many parts of the world. Vitamin deficiencies however, are prevalent in a large number of alcoholics in our country. We have few or no data as to whether mild deficiencies of these vitamins or other nutrients are prevalent in the USA and are responsible for manifestations of ill health.

Extensive nutritional surveys in the USA to evaluate health in relation to nutrient intake have only been undertaken recently, and as of this writing they have been completed in only three states and are in progress in only four or five more. It is important that they be done in many more states to provide factual data on the extent of malnutrition, not only among underprivileged people but also among privileged, and especially among young children. There should be a continued monitoring of the nutritional status of representative groups of our people. Infant mortality rates in the USA are higher than in fifteen other nations and we do not know the contribution of malnutrition to these deaths, but we do know that the death rates are higher among minority groups whose diets tend to be poor.

That there is something wrong with our food distribution system is clear. In the same city it is quite common to find school meals provided in the affluent suburbs but not in the ghetto sections. Food stamps are sometimes available, but frequently the money to buy the stamps is not. Surplus food distribution has been designed much more to help the producer of surplus foods than the poverty stricken consumer.

We do not know how often an empty belly leads individual Americans into crime or what the contribution of anxiety is to violence and rioting in families having insufficient food. We do not yet know the role that malnutrition plays in mental and behavioral development of children.

We do know that all is not well nutritionally in this most affluent of nations. Improved nutrition allied with other measures of health and social justice can make America a better place for all her citizens. It can solve the problems of overnutrition—of too many calories, of too much saturated fat—in the affluent and of nutritional deficiencies and varying degrees of starvation in the poor, the alcoholics, the senile and the dejected.

Interest in nutrition as an important environmental factor in the health of man is increasing and rapidly. This stems from many directions, such as the realization that tooth decay, one of our most prevalent diseases, can be reduced by half or more via the adjustment (usually upward) of the mineral nutrient fluoride in community waters, a process known as fluoridation; that lowering the cholesterol level of the blood lessens the chances of developing coronary heart disease or a stroke; that essential hypertension can frequently be treated simply by a modest loss of weight and a generous decrease in the intake of sodium; that iron deficiency anemia is prevalent in about one-fourth of our total population. It is a noted fact that obesity is widely prevalent in our country and that while by itself and when only moderate it may not be a health hazard, yet it seldom exists by itself and then it is a real hazard to health; and finally the most devastating knowledge is that serious starvation as a partner of poverty is far more prevalent than had been expected.

This manual is not a textbook of nutrition. Several areas of medicine where nutrition is of importance such as diabetes, have been omitted because there already are excellent manuals on the nutritional aspects of these subjects or good chapters in standard medical texts. This is simply a manual on nutrition designed to interest the medical student and others interested in nutrition about the health of man today.

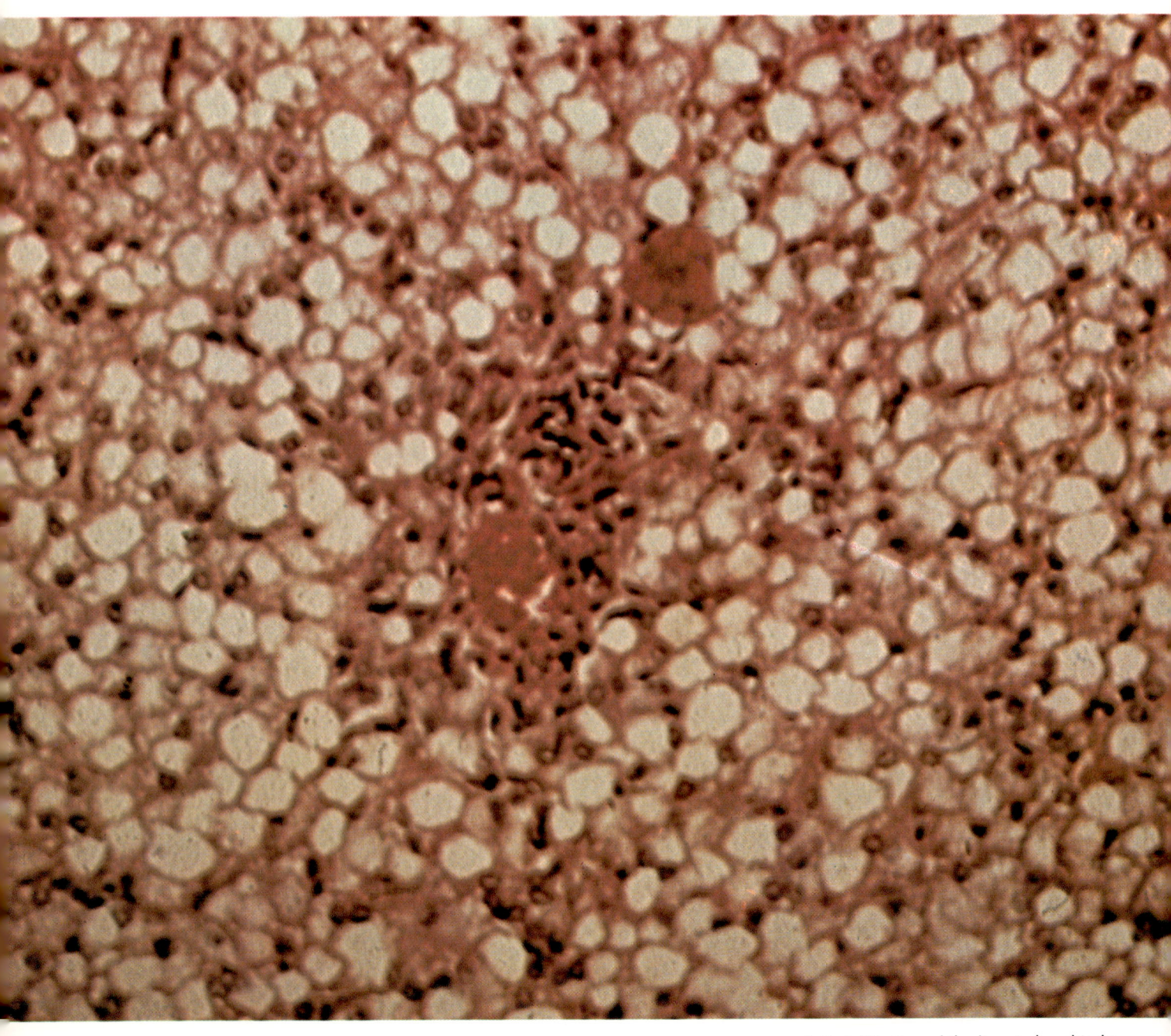

Fatty infiltration of the liver in kwashiorkor.
Michael C. Latham, M.D.
Professor of International Nutrition
Cornell University, Ithaca, New York

Recommended Dietary Allowances of Nutrients

This manual has been prepared primarily for use by medical students and physicians in the United States. Following is part of the introduction to the publication, Recommended Dietary Allowances,[1] which is a report of the Food and Nutrition Board, National Academy of Sciences — National Research Council of the United States. This publication provides the recommended daily dietary allowances of nutrients and gives an explanation of how these allowances are estimated.

"Since 1940, the Food and Nutrition Board has developed formulations of daily nutrient intakes which were judged to be adequate for the maintenance of good nutrition in the population of the United States. These formulations were designated 'Recommended Dietary Allowances' in order to indicate that they were value-judgments based on the existing knowledge of nutritional science and subject to revision as new knowledge became available. The allowances are intended to serve as goals toward which to aim in planning food supplies and as guides for the interpretation of food consumption records of groups of people. Actual nutritional status of groups of people or individuals must be judged on the basis of physical, biochemical, and clinical observations combined with observations on food or nutrient intakes. If the recommended allowances are used as reference standards for interpreting records of food consumption, it should not be assumed that food practices are necessarily poor or that malnutrition exists because the recommendations are not completely met.

"The first edition of Recommended Dietary Allowances was published in 1943. The allowances recommended are those which, in the opinion of the Food and Nutrition Board, will maintain good nutrition in essentially all healthy persons in the United States under current conditions of living.

"The physiological and biochemical bases for the recommended allowances of each specific nutrient are described in the text. For proper understanding, application, and interpretation of the recommended allowances, it is necessary to appreciate how the allowances are related to estimates of average physiological requirements.

"The allowances are designed to afford a margin of sufficiency above average physiological requirements to cover variations among essentially all individuals in the general population. They provide a buffer against the increased needs during common stresses and permit full realization of growth and productive potential; but they are not to be considered adequate to meet additional requirements of persons depleted by disease or traumatic stresses. On the other hand, the allowances are generous with respect to temporary emergency feeding of large groups under conditions of limited food supply and physical disaster.

---

1. *Recommended Dietary Allowances*, 7th Edition, NAS-NRC, Publication 1694, Washington, D.C., 1968.

"The margin of sufficiency above normal physiological requirements is different for each nutrient because of differences in the body storage capacity, in the range of individual requirements, in the precision of assessing requirements, and in the possible hazard of excessive intake of certain nutrients.

"Patterns of food consumption and food supplies in the United States permit ready adaptation to and compliance with the recommended allowances. The final objective of the recommended allowances is to permit and to encourage the development of food practices by the population of the United States that will allow for greatest dividends in health and in disease prevention."

The recommended dietary allowances therefore provide guidelines for the evaluation and development of diets for people in the United States. It should be clearly understood that the values presented are not requirements since many individuals are known to consume smaller amounts than those listed and still enjoy good health. On the other hand it is recognized that the actual requirement is not precisely known for any nutrient and the experimental estimates of requirements always show rather large differences in different experiments and in different individuals. The cause of these variations is generally unknown. No doubt they are partially explained by technical differences or errors of measurement and partly by actual differences in requirements among individuals which may be of genetic origin. When the true requirement is unknown, there is safety in recommending levels of nutrient intake above the estimated minimal need. The recommended dietary allowances therefore must not be considered actual requirements but rather levels of intake which should be entirely adequate for essentially all members of the population. This kind of dietary guidance seems appropriate in an affluent country such as the United States. It may not be appropriate in many parts of the world where more urgent problems exist and where food and money are more limiting factors for many people.

The presentation of one figure as a recommended intake for a particular group as in table I is likely to be somewhat misleading and often misinterpreted. The publication from which it is taken[2] provides explanations and justifications for values presented. The text should be consulted by those who are using the table.

It should be pointed out that the Recommended Dietary Allowances in the various editions are not the same, and never have been, as the Minimum Daily Requirements set forth by the Food and Drug Administration. The latter were usual many years ago in an attempt to try and actually maintain minimum daily requirements. They are now completely out of date, with no evidence to justify their continued use; nevertheless they are still being used by the FDA and therefore by industry.

2. *Recommended Dietary Allowances,* 7th Edition, NAS-NRC, Publication 1694, Washington, D.C.,1968.

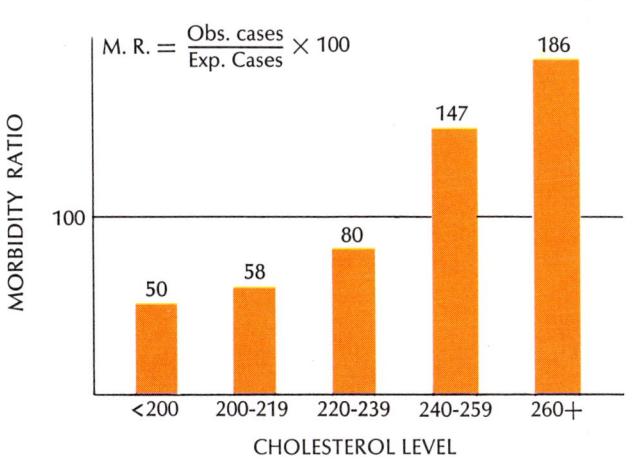

Chart 1a
Relative Risks of Developing Coronary Heart Disease According to Initial Serum Cholesterol Levels men initially aged 30-59 years and followed up for 10 years.

Chart 1b

NUMBER ONE KILLER — 1968

1. Analysis of Causes of Deaths

a. Arteriosclerosis deaths
   Ischemic heart disease 677,260
   Chronic disease of endocardium &
   other myocardial insufficiency 7,630
   Cerebrovascular disease 209,420
   Arteriosclerosis 33,350
                                            927,660

b. Hypertension deaths
   Hypertension heart disease 10,000
   Hypertensive heart & renal disease 7,600
   Hypertension 8,980
                                            26,580

   Total arteriosclerosis and
   hypertension deaths 954,240

c. Deaths from other cardiovascular diseases
   Acute rheumatic fever & chronic
   rheumatic heart disease 16,440
   All other forms of heart disease .. 26,430
   Other diseases of arteries,
   arterioles and capillaries 24,270
                                            67,140

   Total estimated deaths,
   cardiovascular diseases, 1968 1,021,380
   Total estimated deaths,
   all causes, 1968 1,923,000

2. 49.6% of All Deaths in 1968 Were Caused by Arteriosclerosis and Hypertension. Cardiovascular Diseases, as a Whole, Accounted for Over 53% of all Deaths.

Adapted from compilation of the National Health Education Committee, Inc., New York, N. Y. 10017

---

carry out a controlled clinical trial designed to assess risk of disease in an appropriately sampled group in whom a factor associated with risk has been manipulated. A suitable study design, properly controlled is mandatory.

Of all the factors related to atherosclerotic vascular diseases, dietary changes to reduce blood lipids are more practical and effective than is intervention in other risk factors considering the lamentable status of our ability to motivate people to alter their life style. Persistent weight reduction, alteration of smoking habits, changing patterns of physical activity are very difficult to achieve in most individuals. Today there is increasingly secure evidence from clinical trials that dietary changes aimed at reducing the levels of serum lipids, especially cholesterol, can significantly reduce the incidence of coronary heart disease in man. One such study, a longitudinal evaluation of approximately 1,000 high risk individuals whose average serum cholesterol was reduced by 12% through diet alone has shown a significant reduction in coronary heart disease compared to a matched control group.[3] Another controlled trial,[4] using men who had survived a myocardial infarction, has shown that the group treated with a lipid controlled diet had a significantly reduced incidence of myocardial re-infarction and angina pectoris over a five-year follow-up period compared to the counterpart control group. The average reduction in serum cholesterol in the diet-controlled groups was 17%.

3. Christakis, G. et al., *Am. J. Pub. Health* 56:299, 1966.
4. Leren, P., *Acta Med. Scand.*, Suppl. 466, 1966.

The aims of dietary management for the reduction of serum cholesterol are threefold:

1. To lower the intake of saturated fat. The principal sources of saturated fat in the usual diet are from meats and dairy products. A lowered intake can be achieved by the careful selection and trimming of meats and by emphasizing the increased use of fish and poultry which are naturally low in their content of saturated fat. Low fat dairy products–skimmed milk, low fat milks, cottage cheeses, sherbets–can be substituted for their high fat counterparts. The use of high fat baked products, including snacks, should be lessened unless the fat is a polyunsaturated fat.

2. To raise the intake of polyunsaturated fats. These are found in abundance in safflower, corn, soya, and cottonseed oils. Margarines, salad, cooking oils and shortenings made with these oils offer a substitute for animal fats which will maintain the daily fat intake at palatably high levels and contribute to a reduction in serum cholesterol.

3. To lower the intake of dietary cholesterol. The usual dietary intake of 600 to 800 mg. per day can be cut in half by limiting the use of egg yolks to two or three per week. Lessening the consumption of organ meats such as liver and shell fish and increasing the use of leaner meats and lower fat dairy products will also help to limit the cholesterol intake.

Following these guidelines will lead to a modest reduction in the overall level of daily fat calories, from the 40 to 45% in usual diets to a level of 35 to 40%; the ratio of polyunsaturated to saturated fat will be raised to 1:1 or higher.

Another important aspect is that the calorie balance[5] be adjusted to insure a desirable weight; modest restriction of caloric intake and modest increases in the level of physical activity will achieve this.

NOTE ON CIRCULATING LIPIDS

The beta lipoproteins (complexes of triglyceride, cholesterol, and phospholipid wrapped in carrier protein) are the agents most closely associated with atherosclerosis–both in laboratory animals and in man. The measurements of total plasma cholesterol and of fasting triglyceride provide useful though indirect estimates of the level of the beta lipoproteins. While knowledge of cholesterol and triglyceride alone is sufficient for screening and for assessing management in the great proportion of the population, among the 5 per cent of middle-aged individuals with a plasma cholesterol of 300 mg. per 100 ml. or above or with a lactescent fasting serum, determination of electrophoretic or physical-chemical properties of the lipoproteins[6] is important to their management.

5. The American Heart Association, 44 East 23rd Street, New York, New York 10010 has available additional information on modified fat diets.
6. Fredrickson, D. S., Levy, R. I., and Lees, R. S., *New Eng. J. Med.* 276:34, 94, 148, 215, 273, 1967.

II. NUTRITIONAL THERAPY OF CONGESTIVE HEART FAILURE AND HYPERTENSION

Reduction of body sodium by dietary restriction and pharmacologic intervention are the aims of current nutritional therapy of heart failure and hypertension. Net body loss of sodium in the individual with a failing heart reduces extracellular fluid volume, correcting edema and its complications, and reducing circulating fluid volume, all lessening the work of the heart. The resulting improvement of organ perfusion, especially of the kidneys, results in the ability of intrinsic homeostatic mechanisms to regain control of sodium balance, and improves exercise tolerance.

Today's physician is becoming increasingly aware that the natriuretic drugs, the diuretics and cardiac glycosides, are not without hazard, and, lamentably, not infrequently have had fatal consequences. Effective diuretics are associated with potassium as well as sodium loss. Potassium depletion secondary to diuretic therapy increases myocardial irritability and predisposes to threatening arrhythmias. This compromise is potentiated by the cardiac glycosides, drugs used frequently in combination with the potassium-depleting diuretics. Too frequently drugs are employed in the treatment of patients who would respond to dietary sodium restriction alone, if prescribed with the same conviction.

The aim of nutritional therapy is to induce negative sodium balance in the body. The physician prescribes a diet which is adequate nutritionally but restricted in its sodium content. Usual sodium ion intake for an American has been estimated at 3-7 gm. or 150-300 mEq. per day. Therapeutic regimens range from the "no added salt diet," approximately 2.3 gm. sodium (100 mEq./Na.), to as low as 230 mg. sodium (10 mEq.) per day.

Patients frequently misunderstand the sources of salt or sodium in the diet. It should be the responsibility of the physician to insure that the patient understands that foods *naturally* contain sodium. The most understandable explanation is that just as we retain sodium in our bodies, so does the animal, and therefore foods of animal origin—meat, milk, cheese and butter— are major sources of dietary sodium. The processes of preservation of foods often necessitate the addition of salt, and thus many smoked, cured and canned foods contain high concentrations of sodium. Many food condiments and flavor enhancers contain sodium in the form of monosodium glutamate (MSG). Food tables are available which provide information on the amount of sodium contained in common foods, expressed usually in milligrams [with 1 mEq. equal to 23 mg.Na.(Appendix A)]. (The American Heart Association can provide the physician with excellent materials for patient distribution.)

It is true that diuretics and cardiac glycosides are among our most potent therapeutic tools in dealing with a patient with heart failure, and are definitely indicated in addition to dietary sodium restriction in the severely compromised patient. If there exists a clinical necessity for the use of these drugs together, or of the diuretics alone, potassium supplementation must be instituted. Potassium salts are gastric irritants and are unpalatable, causing nausea, vomiting, and rejection by the patient. This is why potassium salts have been given as enteric coated tablets. This preparation may cause ulceration of the small intestine and its unhappy consequences. If potassium supplementation is necessary, potassium-rich foods are an economical, palatable, and a simple approach contrasted with potassium elixers. Especially with these preparations the possibility of overdosage must be considered, another probable fatal result of the failure to recognize the safer nutritional approach.

Patients on diuretic therapy may require potassium ion intakes as high as 5 gm. (130 mEq.) per day. A list of foods which contain concentrated amounts of potassium is found in Appendix A. The nutritional approach to sodium restriction and potassium supplementation cannot be understated as important adjuncts for the patient requiring manipulation of electrolyte balance.

Obesity

A type of malnutrition which is highly prevalent and readily visible, is obesity, the by-product of affluence and of a way of life in which the levels of caloric intake and energy expenditure are unbalanced. Aside from the often serious social and psychological stigma created by obesity, it is also associated with an increased risk of many diseases and of aggravating others; gross obesity generally shortens the life span itself. Cardiovascular and pulmonary diseases, hypertension, diabetes, cholelithiasis, peripheral vascular and orthopedic disorders are among the medical hazards linked to or aggravated by adiposity. Within the present capacity of the physician, the treatment of obesity is often discouraging. It is the nature of obesity to perpetuate itself. Thus, it may well be that *prevention* of excessive weight gain will offer the most effective and practical approach to the problem.

Figure 1
Triceps skinfold thickness measured by a skinfold caliper. The tissue on both arms should be measured to obtain an average measurement of adipose tissue.

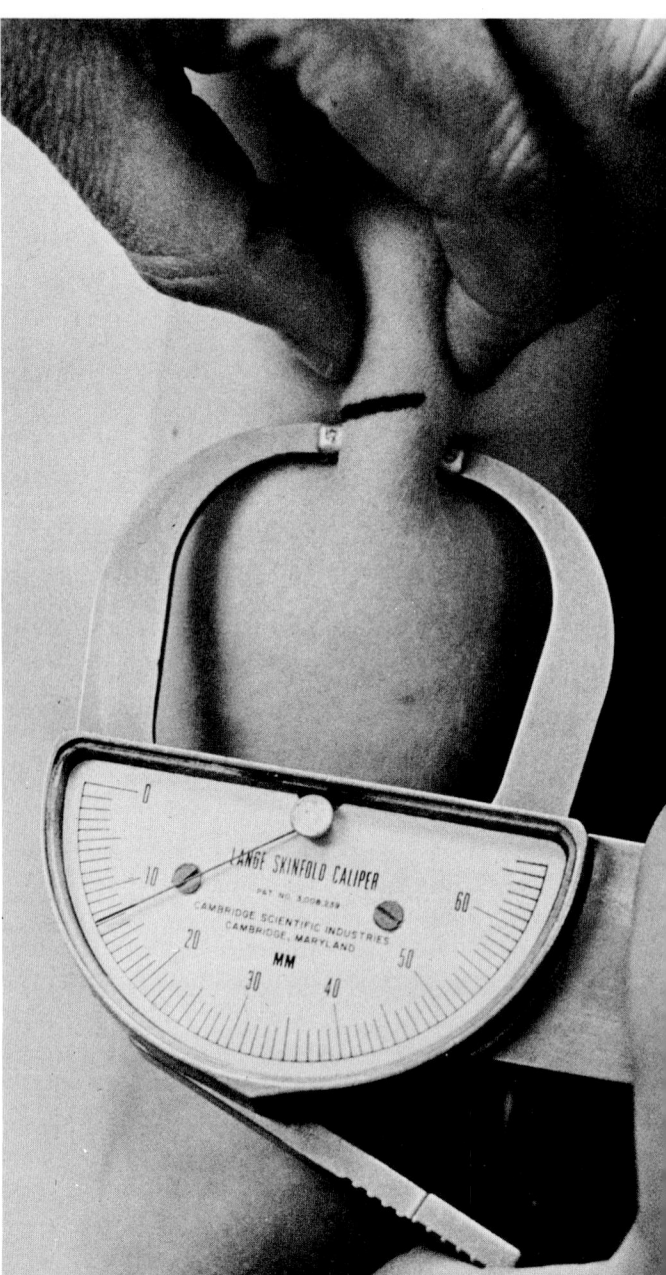

Definitions and Assessment

The terms obesity and overweight are not synonymous; the former denotes an excess of adipose tissue; the latter makes no distinction among the several body components, muscle, bone, or fat. Body fluid is not considered. An individual may be overweight relative to some arbitrary standard and yet not be obese. While football players are the classically cited examples of this, such instances are not often found among the general, middle-aged population. By measuring weight for height and comparing this to standards approximate to sex and age, one is not necessarily able to qualify an individual on the continuum of adiposity. Gross overweight usually implies gross obesity; such individuals clearly have a risk of increased morbidity and mortality from major diseases. But the relative risks of lesser degrees of overweight are not clear and it is probably the measurement of adiposity that is relevant in this regard.

Total adipose tissue cannot be conveniently or directly measured, but the determination of skinfold thickness at standard sites does offer a simple method for quantitating adiposity. Such estimates are highly correlated with total body fat; constant pressure skinfold calipers allow the physician to make these measurements reliably. The triceps and subscapular skinfolds are the sites generally used. The former is more easily obtained and gives more reproducible results. With the right arm flexed at 90°, a tape measure is used to accurately locate on the back of the triceps the midpoint between tip of the acromion and olecranon. The caliper is applied to the fold of skin pulled away at this location. Upper limits of normal values for a healthy Caucasian American population are shown in Appendix D.

Height-weight tables have been the most commonly used standards for quantitating overnutrition; their limitations have already been mentioned. The tables of desirable or ideal weight (for sex and weight) represent those weights of insurees with optimal mortality experience (Appendix D). For many obese middle-aged patients, these weights represent goals which are discouragingly beyond achieving.

Height, weight, skinfold thickness, an appraisal of an individual's general appearance, an evaluation of his own motivation and goals provide the basis for a meaningful evaluation of obesity and for a realistic attempt at a successful treatment.

Among women, increases in adipose tissue are most marked during pregnancies and after the menopause. Males tend to acquire adipose tissue at a more constant rate from the third decade onward. Obese children and adolescents are a major reservoir for relatively intractable obesity in adult life; they usually have much more difficulty in achieving and maintaining weight reduction as adults.

Treatment and Prevention

The difficulties encountered with treatment strongly suggest a concern for the *prevention* of obesity. The major focus on preventive measures ought to be in adolescence and early adulthood. The long term aim of either treatment or prevention is to instill a sensible program of dietary *and exercise* habits which will assure stable energy balance throughout life.

Diet

A proper therapeutic diet for obesity should provide all necessary nutrients in sufficient amounts and be restricted in caloric content. It should be palatable and easily available from the viewpoint of economics and convenience. The patient should be educated so that once desired weight has been achieved, minor changes, such as increasing portion size of foods allowed, will provide a proper maintenance diet. The caloric deficit desired can be estimated from the fact that a pound of body fat respresents the equivalent of about 3500 calories. Thus a daily deficit of 500 calories will lead to an average weekly loss of one pound. In relatively active patients, a daily intake of less than 1500 calories for men and 1000 for women is poorly tolerated. Increased physical activity can help increase the caloric deficit so that a patient can obtain a total deficit of 500 calories per day without cutting food intake to this extent. Thus a decrease in calories from food and drink of 300 per day and an increase in caloric expenditure of 200 calories per day will accomplish the same effect as a decrease of 500 calories in the diet and be more acceptable to most people.

Experience has shown that a balanced diet with 12-14 per cent of calories as protein, 35 to 40 per cent in fat calories, a reduction in saturated fats, with the remaining calories supplied by carbohydrate, all provided by foods of sufficient variety, is the best diet over a long period of time. There is no evidence that more extreme diets, especially fad diets, which constantly appear and/or disappear have any advantage over a calorically restricted, balanced, "normal" diet. Moreover fad diets do not provide realistic programs which can be followed for the necessary period of time needed to maintain body weight, and some of them are actually dangerous to health.

The chief advantage of "formula diets" which became popular during the past decade is that they provide a simple, rigid regimen that does not need to be based on any knowledge of food and food values. They may be useful at the beginning of a weight control program or for a one-meal a day replacement in certain instances.

Bulk-producing agents such as methyl cellulose have not been shown to be of any special merit. Salads, fruits and vegetables are superior bulk-producing agents as well as being more palatable and more likely to become part of a lifelong dietary pattern.

Salt restriction is useful in obese subjects with a tendency to excessive fluid retention, particularly middle-aged and older women and sedentary persons. Salt restriction is a more sound measure than the use of diuretics to prevent excessive water retention.

Most appetite-depressant drugs are sympathomimetic amines related in structure to amphetamine. They act chiefly by stimulating the ventromedial (satiety) hypothalamic center, but may have other accessory actions, including stimulation of spontaneous physical activity and of free fatty acid release by adipose tissue. In most cases, the effective duration of amphetamine treatment is of the order of a month to six weeks. They are useful to tide a patient over periods of excessive hunger that persist in spite of meal and snack adjustment. Anorexigenic agents are most useful at the onset of treatment and with patients who have recently become obese.

Dessicated thyroid has been used as an adjunct to weight reduction on the grounds that obese patients are in a hypometabolic state and, therefore, can lose weight easier if metabolic stimulation is accomplished. Most obese patients, however, are euthyroid. Thyroid hormones in small doses suppress endogenous hormone production, resulting in no net effect. Larger doses produce a hyperthyroid state with its serious side effects, and cause loss of lean body mass rather than fat. The drug is not recommended for general use in weight reduction programs.

Repeated cycles of weight changes are an all too frequent result of crash programs and fad diets. Such cycles may be more harmful than the maintenance of a steady weight, even at levels of moderate obesity.

Exercise is a most important factor in a realistic reducing program. For most individuals, exercise is the great variable in energy expenditure, and reduction or elimination of exercise is not generally followed by a reduction in food intake. Conversely, exercise does not increase voluntary food intake in inactive subjects until it has reached a certain critical duration and intensity.

In general, the long-term results of a variety of weight reduction programs utilizing both individual and group approaches to weight control have been unhappily discouraging. Characteristically, once desired weight was achieved, therapy ceased, and weight was regained. Because maintenance of the new desirable weight requires a new pattern of eating and activity for the individual, it is highly probable that intermittent support following weight loss might prevent the common return to pre-dieting weight levels.

For further reading on the subject of obesity consult: U.S. Department of Health, Education and Welfare, U.S. Public Health Service's booklet on, "Obesity and Health," available from U.S. Government Printing Office, Washington, D.C. 20402.

Dental Caries

Dental caries is the most widespread disease in the United States. In some parts of the country as many as 90 per cent of the population surveyed have serious dental problems requiring either tooth extraction or filling. A complete loss of teeth as early as adolescence is occasionally seen and by middle age is fairly common. Edentulous persons often have difficulty in consuming certain foods and this sometimes makes it hard for them to get a balanced diet. The dental profession does not have the trained manpower to provide adequate dental care to everyone. If poverty and lack of knowledge were not important factors in limiting the numbers seeking dental treatment then dentists would be overwhelmed and quite unable to cope with the dental pathology that would be presented to them. The prevention of dental caries by whatever means possible is therefore of great public health importance.

That modern western diets have had an effect on the prevalence of dental caries is shown by the much higher number of teeth that are decayed, missing and filled in groups of persons of the same age that are surveyed in say Africa and the United States. It is al-

On The Way to Better Health

Figure 4a
Mealtime for hospitalized children in New Guinea.

Figure 4b
School lunch in a village in Tunisia.

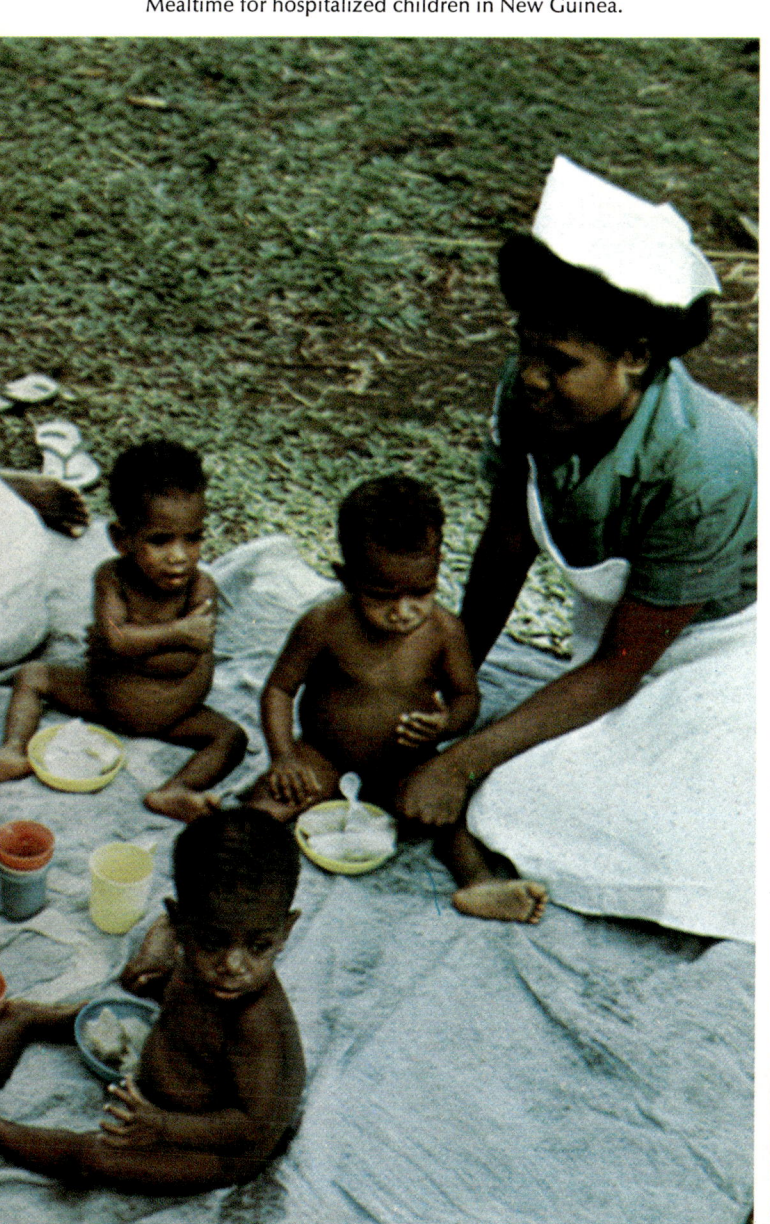
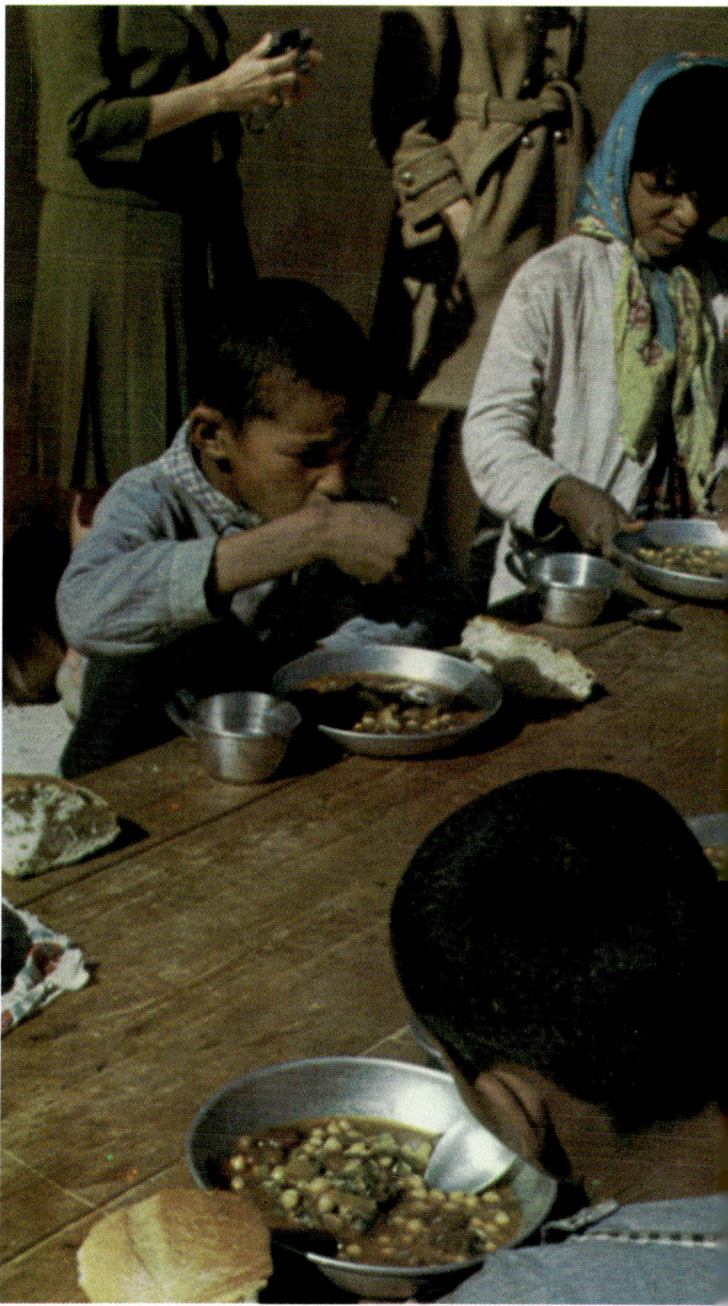

KWASHIORKOR
Etiology and Epidemiology

Kwashiorkor occurs mainly in children 1 to 3 years of age. It is common in many developing countries of Asia, Africa and Latin America, but has been reported in Europe and the United States where it is associated with poverty.

The disease occurs in children whose diet is grossly deficient in protein. Often the food that the child is receiving is of a type which contains mainly carbohydrate and little protein. In many parts of the world it is a disease of the weaning period when the child is taken from the breast onto a mainly starchy diet. An adequate intake of breast milk will provide a satisfactory diet for the first four to six months of an infant's life. After that, mainly because of reduced quantities, breast milk provides merely a useful protein-rich dietary supplement to whatever other food the child is receiving.

Important factors often implicated in the complex etiology of kwashiorkor are:

(a) The rapid growth and relatively high protein requirements of the rapidly growing young child.

(b) A protein-poor, staple food for the child, e.g., manioc, bananas, sugar.

(c) Poor infant feeding practices.

(d) A lack of protein-rich foods both animal (meat, milk, fish, eggs, etc.) and vegetable (e.g., beans, peanuts, etc.).

(e) A poor distribution of available food in the family (e.g., the adults and older children often get the major share of protein-rich foods such as meat.).

(f) Seasonal food shortages.

(g) Poverty and its attendant ills.

(h) Cultural dietary practices including food taboos which may preclude the child consuming certain available and desirable foods.

(i) Infections such as diarrhea, measles, whooping cough, etc.

(j) Ignorance or lack of knowledge on the part of parents or guardians, on what foods are needed in the child's diet.

(k) Psychological factors which may affect the appetite of the child.

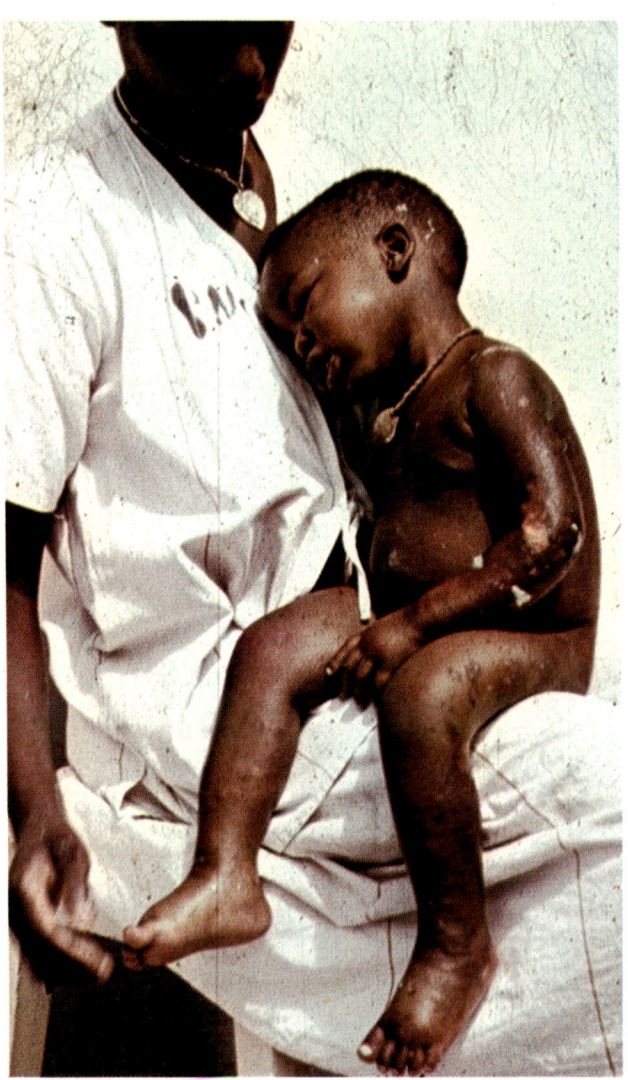

Figure 3b
Kwashiorkor in an African child showing edema and dermatosis.

with iron, but only in small amounts. The quantity should be increased as much as possible without interfering with the flavor. However, women and girls do not ordinarily consume large amounts of bread. Thus foods other than bread that can be suitably fortified with iron should be found.

Control of iron deficiency in the United States is complicated by the fact that total food intake becomes smaller as the population becomes more and more sedentary and many girls and women are excessively concerned about obesity. When the total caloric intake is low and approximately 40% of the calories are supplied as fat and 20-25% as sugar, there is little room in the diet for iron-containing foods. Improved manufacturing methods, use of stainless and aluminum utensils and emphasis on cleanliness have lowered the total iron intake.

Protein-Calorie Malnutrition of Young Children

Protein-calorie malnutrition in young children constitutes the most important and widespread nutritional problem in the world today. The two main clinical syndromes are kwashiorkor and nutritional marasmus. In kwashiorkor the principal deficiency is of protein whereas in marasmus there is an overall deficit in food intake including calories and protein. From the clinical point of view there are many intermediate cases which are difficult to fit into either category and which have some of the symptoms and signs of both conditions.

It should be recalled that these clinical entities constitute only the relatively small exposed part of the enormous iceberg of protein-calorie malnutrition. There are perhaps 99 children who are receiving an inadequate diet, who are poorly grown and who are prone to infections for every frank case of serious clinical protein-calorie deficiency disease. These 99 children are mild or sub-clinical cases of protein-calorie malnutrition, and typically remain submerged in the population of children. They are liable to be precipitated into one of these clinical states by any of a variety of causes.

Over the past two decades kwashiorkor has been recognized and studied in many parts of the world. It is now accepted as one disease with a few local variations. During this period, the emphasis has been on protein deficiency and a world-wide effort has been made to increase the quantity and quality of protein available to children. More recently attention has turned to the equal importance of a shortage of calories as part of an overall deficiency of food in the diets of young children.

Kwashiorkor and nutritional marasmus can be regarded as the two extremes of protein-calorie malnutrition of young children. However, very many cases of protein-calorie malnutrition are intermediate and this has given rise to such names as "marasmic-kwashiorkor" in cases where kwashiorkor is superimposed on marasmus. A separate description is given kwashiorkor and of nutritional marasmus, but the clinician must expect many cases to be intermediate between the two extremes.

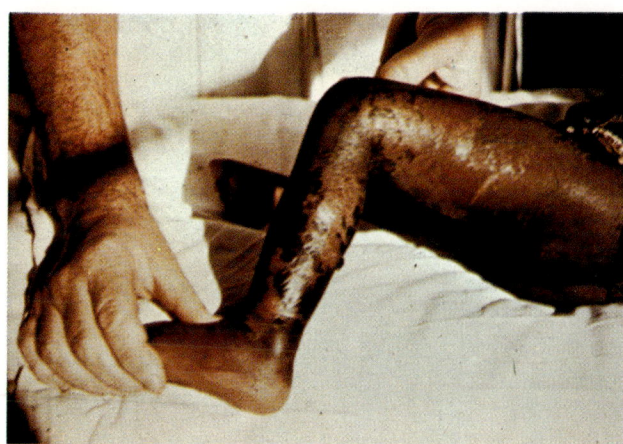

Figure 3a
Kwashiorkor—skin lesions.

Iron Deficiency Anemia

Iron deficiency is one of the most common nutritional deficiencies in the United States. It occurs most frequently in infants beyond 6 months of age, in adolescent girls, and in women in the reproductive period. While good data on prevalence of iron deficiency in any group are not available, it is known to be high in some segments of the population. There are difficulties in defining iron deficiency. Presumably the sequence of events during iron depletion would be loss of iron stores (which may be estimated by staining marrow smears for iron), fall in plasma iron (normal = 50 μg./100 ml.), increase in iron-binding capacity of plasma (normally over 10% saturation), and, finally, development of anemia. In severe iron deficiency this is usually a hypochromic microcytic anemia. The frequency with which iron deficiency is encountered will depend upon the criteria used. Most often simple measurement of hemoglobin or hematocrit has been used. This will certainly underestimate the extent of iron depletion.

Iron is absorbed and excreted only with difficulty. In the usual adult male, 0.5 to 1.0 mg. of iron is lost daily. In the adult menstruating woman, the usual losses are twice as high, often even more, depending upon the amount of blood loss. Similarly, there appears to be great variation in the ability of individuals to absorb dietary iron. On the average, about 10% of the dietary iron is absorbed. An intake of 10 mg. of iron per day would be required to replace the loss of 1 mg. in the adult male and greater in the adult female. The situation is further complicated by the accumulating data showing that the availability of iron in foods may vary greatly. It has been reported that iron in wheat is poorly absorbed whereas that in meat is well absorbed. These differences might, however, be modified by the mixture of foods consumed.

A recent report indicated that egg yolk impairs the absorption of iron, this despite the fact that it is one of the better food sources of iron.[13]

In the adult, iron deficiency is frequently associated with blood loss. In many parts of the world excessive blood losses are associated with hookworm infestation, leading to serious iron deficiency anemia. High iron requirements are also associated with growth, iron being required for all cells and particularly for the increase in blood volume. Iron deficiency is frequently encountered in infancy, especially in infants born to anemic mothers. The normal infant is born with iron stores but milk is a very poor source of iron. Unless supplemented foods, rich in iron or supplements containing iron are provided, anemia will be common in the latter part of infancy and early childhood. Anemia and iron depletion may also be common in adolescent girls who bear the combined stress of growth and menstruation. Pregnancy also imposes the stress of the growth of the fetus combined with an expansion of the blood volume. With poor dietary habits, young girls and women may often enter pregnancy with reduced iron stores.

With large variations in iron requirements and in iron utilization, it is obviously difficult to estimate the iron requirement of any individual. The Recommended Dietary Allowances are deliberately set toward the high side so that the needs of the majority will be met at these levels. However, the new allowances (1968) specify higher levels for women than previously and these levels will apparently not be met by the usual diets in the United States. The question is therefore posed, should the usual diet contain enough iron to meet the needs of individuals with high iron requirements? If so, how can this be accomplished? Most bread and flour in the United States is now fortified

---

13. Symposium: Iron Deficiency and Absorption, *Am. J. Clin. Nutr.* 21:1138, 1968.

Osteoporosis

Osteoporosis is a chronic disease of aging. It is extremely prevalent in the United States and as the population tends to live longer it is becoming ever more important.

The disease is characterized by an excessive demineralization of bone which is often responsible for considerable pain. This is commonly in the back and may radiate around the trunk and extend into the legs. It sometimes incapacitates the individual because the pain is aggravated by movement and by jarring the spine in walking. A frequent complication in the elderly is the fracturing of bones. This may be the collapse of one or more vertebrae, it may be the fracture of the hip due to a minor fall, or it may involve some other bone.

Osteoporosis is usually diagnosed radiologically. A good radiograph of the spine may be helpful but for survey purposes x-rays of the hand, wrist or jaw are more useful. There is in these areas less variability due to soft tissue and gas overlay of the bone. In all cases the shadow of the bone shows diminished density.

Full descriptions of osteoporosis appear in the standard medical textbooks. From a nutritional point of view there is new interest in the disease because evidence now indicates that fluoride is effective in the treatment of the disease[9] and may be important also in its prevention. It is known that fluoride becomes a part of the bone substance just as it does in dental enamel, replacing hydroxyl ions in the chemical composition of the bone and giving rise to a larger bone crystal which may be less liable to resorption.

The first evidence that fluoride intake might be an important factor in osteoporosis came from a comparison of x-rays taken in two communities, one of which had water with a low fluoride content and one with a high fluoride content. It was found that in the former community there was substantially more osteoporosis and decreased bone density.[10] A recent study was made in two comparable areas of North Dakota[11] which had differing amounts of fluoride in their water. Judged both by relative bone density and from the presence or absence of collapsed vertebra there was substantially less osteoporosis in the high-fluoride areas.

Fluoride has now been used in the treatment of osteoporosis for a number of years with beneficial results. In treatment, doses have varied from 5 mg. to over 60 mg. of fluoride daily usually given as a sodium fluoride tablet. The daily dose necessary to produce remission is much larger than that which can be ingested from drinking fluoridated water. However, this does not mean that drinking fluoridated water from an early age may not help to substantially reduce osteoporosis in the elderly in the later years. This however remains to be proved.

There was a widely held belief that calcium deficiencies in the diets of the elderly were important in the causation of osteoporosis. This is now disputed[12] as there are no good studies to substantiate such a claim. Calcium has not been effective in the treatment of the disease and there is no sound epidemiological evidence to show that osteoporosis is more prevalent where deficient calcium diets are regularly eaten. In fact, osteoporosis has been shown to be an important problem in the United States, Great Britian and Scandinavia, three areas where calcium intakes tend to be rather high.

9. Bernstein, D. S. and Cohen, P., *J. Clin. Endocrinol.* 27:197, 1967.
10. Leone, N. C. et al., *Arch. Indust. Health* 21:326, 1960.
11. Bernstein, D. S., et al., *JAMA* 198:499, 1966.
12. Hegsted, D. M., *J. Am. Dietet. Assoc.* 50:105, 1967.

than did the children in the other communities.[8] Trials in other cities and in several countries have given similar results. Today there are over 7000 communities serving over 90 million people that have fluoridated water in the United States.

There is no doubt that the fluoridation of water supplies is a public health measure of very great importance. It is the responsibility of every physician to urge and support fluoridation of the water supply of his community where needed. Generally the opponents of fluoridation fall into three categories. They are health faddists, those who for quasi-religious reasons are opposed to any type of medication, and those who equate fluoridation with an interference to their individual rights. Fluoridation has been found to be absolutely safe at one part per million (ppm). Fluoridation is not a form of medication for it is an adjustment of the level of a nutrient just as is the fortification of bread with vitamins. Fluoridation is no more an infringement of freedom of individual rights than is the chlorination of water or the regulation of the speed limit.

There are substitutes for fluoridation such as pills, drops or fluoridated toothpaste but none combine the efficiency, the effectiveness and economy of fluoridation for the mass of the general public. The addition of fluoride to infant vitamin preparations is very useful because fluoride has its maximum effectiveness when received early in life. Such preparations are not contraindicated when fluoridated water is consumed but actually give added protection from dental decay.

8. Shaw, J. H., in *Modern Nutrition in Health and Disease*, edited by Wohl and Goodhart, Lea and Febiger, Philadelphia, 1968.

Chart 5
Incidence of Decayed and Filled Deciduous Teeth
(Three years after first dental examination)
Patient age approximately 7

	Number of Patients	% of Children with All Good Teeth	Mean No. of New Decayed & Filled Teeth
Infant Group (Fluoride-Vitamin from Birth)	108	60.2	0.98
Water Group (Fluoride in Water from Birth)	41	43.9	1.59
Baseline Group (Fluoride-Vitamin since Age 4)	277	30.3	2.14
Control Group (No Fluoride)	212	24.5	2.92

Infants started on fluoride from birth compared to a control group showed more than twice as many children with all good teeth at age seven. These same groups showed approximately one filled tooth in the fluoride group for every three in the child who had no fluoride.

There is a statistical difference ($P < .01$) between the "Control" and "Infant" group and between the "Infant" and "Baseline" group ($P < .01$) with the "Infant" group having a statistically higher percentage of children with all good teeth. $P =$ probability.

Chart 6
Decayed, Missing and Filled Teeth *of children 6-10 years old in fluoridated and non-fluoridated cities*

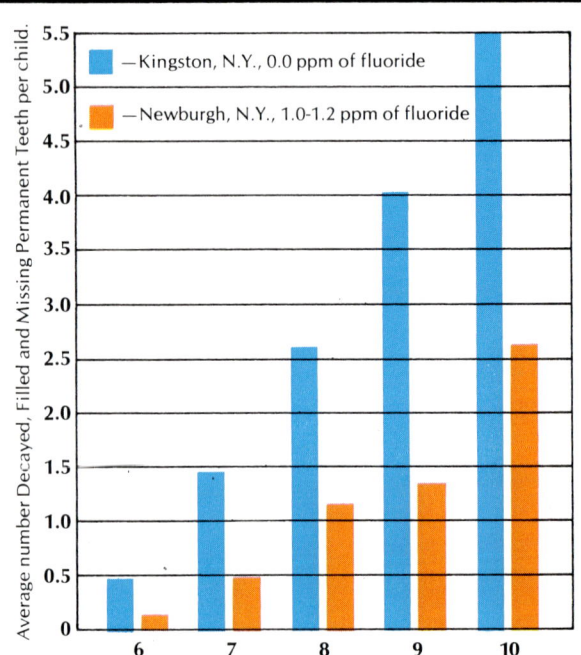

Results from fluoridation in 6-10 year old children in Kingston, N. Y. (no fluoride) and Newburgh, N. Y. (1.0-1.2 ppm of fluoride).

Chart 2
Reduction in Decayed, Missing and Filled Permanent Teeth) *(6 and 7 year-olds, 7 years after fluoridation)*

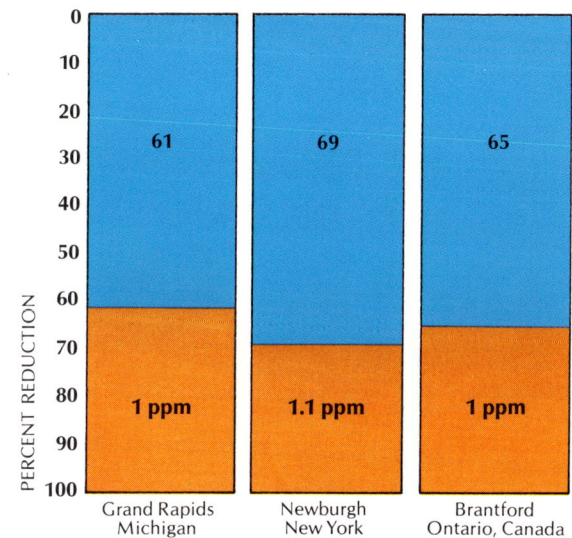

Dental examinations on 6 and 7 year-old children, seven years after the institution of fluoridation, have revealed a reduction of 61%, 69% and 65% in decayed, missing or filled teeth in Grand Rapids, Michigan; Newburgh, New York, and Brantford, Ontario, Canada, respectively.

Chart 4
Interaction of fluoride with the hydroxyapatite mineral lattice of the teeth.

$$3 \cdot Ca_3 P_2 O_8 \cdot Ca(OH)_2 \quad \text{HYDROXYAPATITE}$$
$$+ 2 F^- \quad \text{(caries-susceptible)}$$
$$\downarrow$$
$$3\, Ca_3 P_2 O_8 \cdot Ca(F)_2 \quad \text{FLUORAPATITE}$$
$$+ 2 OH^- \quad \text{(promotes caries-resistance)}$$

Chart 3
Decayed, Missing, and Filled Teeth* per Child
Ten Years After Fluoridation   *Permanent teeth

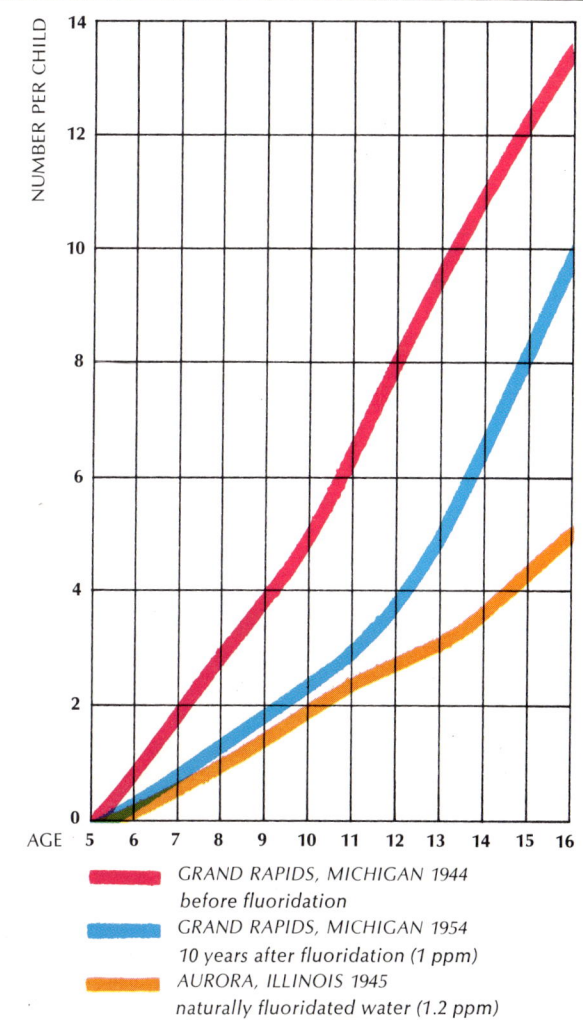

GRAND RAPIDS, MICHIGAN 1944
before fluoridation
GRAND RAPIDS, MICHIGAN 1954
10 years after fluoridation (1 ppm)
AURORA, ILLINOIS 1945
naturally fluoridated water (1.2 ppm)

This chart shows a reduction in dental caries of permanent teeth by 60-70 percent in children who consumed fluoridated water from birth versus those who were denied this important nutrient.

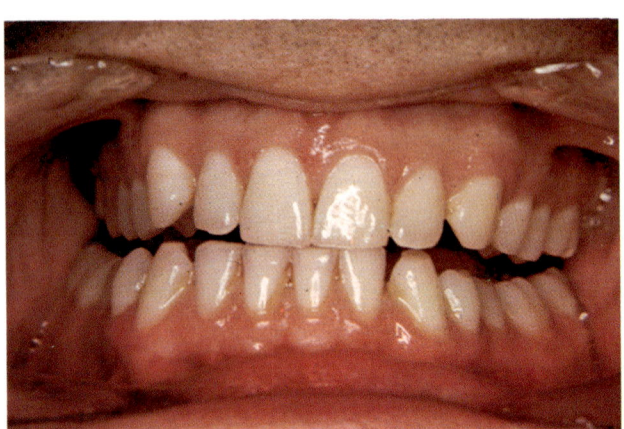

Figure 2a
Male, age 44, drank well water with fluoride content of 1 ppm, no decayed, missing or filled teeth. (DMF/O)

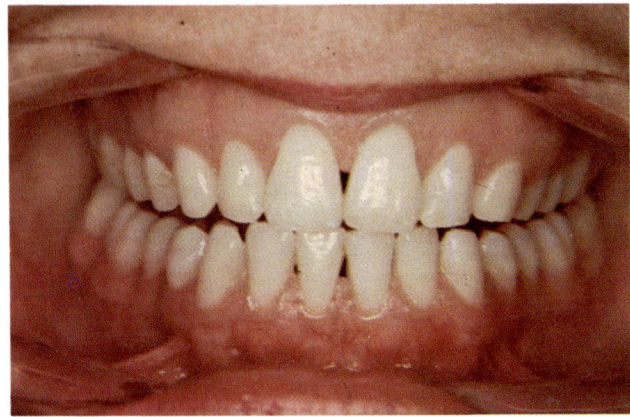

Figure 2b
Female, age 39 (sister of man in Figure 2a). Also has perfect teeth, (DMF/O) drank well water with fluoride content of 1 ppm all her life.

most certain that sticky adherent carbohydrate foods with a low rate of clearance from the oral cavity are an important factor in this respect.[7]

Many nutrients are necessary for the development of the teeth and surrounding structures. Vitamin A is important for normal bone growth. Inadequate growth patterns which result in orthodontic problems can result from vitamin A deficiency. The effects of a deficiency of vitamin C on the soft supporting tissues of the teeth have been described in the section dealing with scurvy. It should be noted that these gum lesions do not occur in the edentulous. Protein is also essential for the normal development of the teeth and supporting tissues.

Vitamin D, calcium and phosphorus which are important in bone development are also essential to the growth of the teeth. There is some controversy as to whether vitamin D supplementation helps to reduce caries-susceptibility. The general balance of evidence suggests that where adequate quantities of vitamin

D, obtained either from the diet or from exposure of the body to sunlight, are absent then vitamin D taken orally will help reduce the caries rate.

However fluoride is the single most important nutrient in relation to dental caries. In the 1930's it was observed that individuals who had access to drinking water that contained 1 to 2 parts per million (ppm) of fluoride had considerably less tooth decay than persons whose water supply had much lower amounts of fluoride. It was subsequently found that in areas where the water had very little fluoride it was possible to reduce the incidence of dental caries by 60 to 70 per cent by adjusting the fluoride level of the water to about 1 ppm. In 1945 a careful experimental trial was begun using three communities (Newburgh, New York; Evanston, Illinois; and Grand Rapids, Michigan) in which fluoride was added to the water. Three neighboring control cities were chosen with no fluoridation and where the fluoride content of the water was low. After ten years it was found that children who had been receiving fluoridated water from an early age had 60 to 70 per cent less dental caries

7. Shaw, J. H., in *Modern Nutrition in Health and Disease*, edited by Wohl and Goodhart, Lea and Febiger, Philadelphia, 1968.

Figure 5
Nutritional marasmus showing extreme wasting in child from Rotterdam, Holland, during World War II.

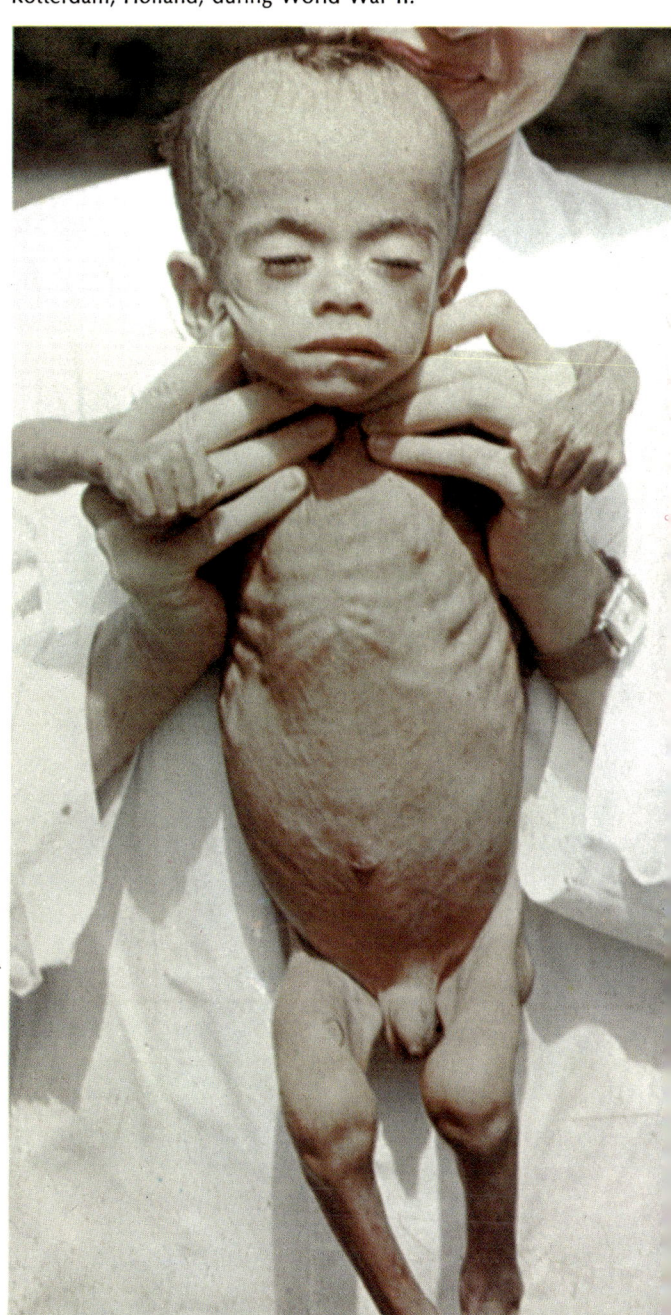

normal. In severe cases the loss of flesh is obvious. The ribs are prominent, the face has a characteristic monkey-like appearance, the limbs are very thin, but the abdomen may be protuberant and in general the child looks like the starved individual which he is.

(b) *Wasting*–The muscles are extremely wasted. There is little if any subcutaneous fat remaining. The skin hangs in wrinkles, especially around the buttocks and thighs.

(c) *Appetite*—Whereas the child with kwashiorkor has anorexia, the child with marasmus frequently has a good appetite. In fact, like any starving creature he may be ravenous, often sucking his hands and clothing.

(d) *Mental state*—Most children with marasmus appear bright eyed and alert. They are not usually disinterested or irritable, like children with kwashiorkor.

(e) *Anemia* is usually present.

(f) *Diarrhea* is common, but is not a constant feature.

An advanced case of nutritional marasmus presents an unmistakable picture. The infant is appallingly thin but the belly in contrast to the rest of the body may be protuberant. The disease, unlike kwashiorkor does not lead to edema or flaky paint dermatosis. Hair changes similar to kwashiorkor can occur, but are less common. Signs of vitamin deficiency, especially of vitamin A, may accompany marasmus.

Laboratory findings

Serum proteins may be reduced, but less so than in kwashiorkor.

The hydroxyproline-creatinine index[14] is low, but the ratio of essential to non-essential amino acids is less altered than in kwashiorkor.

The liver is not infiltrated with fat.

Treatment

Treatment is similar to that described for kwashiorkor, but an adequate intake of calories and protein is mandatory to allow for weight gain and growth.

14. Whitehead, R. G., *Lancet* 2:567, 1965.

gm. of protein per kilogram of body weight per day.

If diarrhea is severe, potassium should be administered at a dose of approximately 0.5 gm. potassium chloride in water three times a day.

Antibiotics should be given to combat infection. In malarial areas, chloroquine or some other antimalarial drug is also desirable.

When shock or severe anemia or dehydration occurs, appropriate supportive measures are indicated. In cases of shock or if the anemia is severe, a blood transfusion might prove life saving. Anemia of a moderate nature can be treated with oral or parenteral iron therapy.

Severe dehydration calls for the administration of intravenous (or intraperitoneal) electrolyte solutions.

Vitamins should be given for vitamin deficiencies and it is especially important to treat any evidence of eye changes caused by vitamin A deficiency.

Severe cases of kwashiorkor can be expected to respond quite rapidly to the above regimen. The diarrhea and gastrointestinal symptoms subside, diuresis occurs with rapid reduction of edema and as the anorexia disappears the mood of the child begins to change and a smile may be a good prognostic sign.

At this stage the treatment can be modified and will be similar for mild cases not requiring hospitalization—consisting of a more varied diet rich in protein. The mother's cooperation in the dietary regimen is important and should form an integral part of therapy, as her nutritional education is expanded.

NUTRITIONAL MARASMUS
Etiology and Epidemiology

Nutritional marasmus is common in nearly all developing countries and in contrast to kwashiorkor is more common in children under 1 year of age, although it is not restricted to this age group. The disease is a form of starvation and therefore the underlying causes are numerous but all involve lack of food and any kind of food. In the United States nutritional marasmus is occasionally seen in grossly neglected children, but may also occur secondary to such diseases as cystic fibrosis, celiac disease or overwhelming infections.

In developing countries a common cause is early cessation of breast feeding. This may be due to death of the mother, failure of lactation, separation of the infant from the mother, or most commonly the mother's desire to feed her infant from the bottle rather than the breast. In this latter event she may be influenced by advertisements and the impact of alien cultures into believing that this is a superior or more sophisticated method of infant feeding. Early cessation of breast feeding does not of course necessarily lead to marasmus. However, a large proportion of people in developing countries do not have sufficient income to purchase enough milk formula to feed a baby properly. As a result the tendency is to overdilute the mixture with water which then fails to provide adequate calories. Similarly few households in these countries have a safe water supply or items in their home which simplify the sterile preparation of bottles of formula for an infant. This combined with a lack of knowledge concerning hygiene commonly leads to the development of gastrointestinal infection which starts the vicious circle leading to marasmus.

Other common causes of marasmus are prematurity, mental deficiency and gastrointestinal disease such as diarrhea or malabsorption. Many of the factors listed under the etiology of kwashiorkor may also be involved.

Nutritional Marasmus

The following are the main features of nutritional marasmus:

(a) *Growth failure*—In all cases there is clear evidence of growth failure. If the age of the child is known the weight will be extremely low by normal standards and the height will also usually be below

The Disease

The following are the main features of kwashiorkor:

(a) *Growth failure* which is always present. If the child's age is known he will be found to be shorter, and except in cases with gross edema, lighter than normal.

(b) *Wasting* is always a feature, but may be masked by edema. The wasting is often evident in the muscles of the arms and legs.

(c) *Edema* always occurs and is a most important feature of the disease. It may affect any part of the body. In an ambulant child it usually starts as a slight swelling of the feet which often spreads up the legs. Later the hands, scrotum and face may all be affected.

(d) *Mental changes* are invariably present. The child is usually apathetic and disinterested in his surroundings. At the same time he is miserable and irritable when being moved or disturbed. He is unsmiling and his behavioral development is retarded.

(e) *Hair changes*—In kwashiorkor the hair often shows changes in texture, in color, in strength, and in ease of pluckability. The tight curl of African or Afro-American hair is often lost, the hair becomes silkier and loses its lustre. Black hair becomes brown or reddish brown in color. In Latin America parallel strips of discolored hair have been labeled the "flag sign."

(f) *Skin changes*—These are not invariable, but if present may be very characteristic. The skin, especially of the face, may show depigmentation. In some cases a dermatosis develops especially in areas of friction such as the groins and behind the knees. Darkly pigmented patches appear and these may desquamate like old blistered paint, which has given rise to the term "flaky paint dermatosis." Beneath the flakes are atrophic areas which may resemble a healing burn.

(g) *Diarrhea*—Stools are frequently loose and contain undigested particles of food. Sometimes they are offensive, watery and blood-stained.

(h) *Anemia*—Most cases of kwashiorkor have some degree of anemia. This is due in part to a lack of protein to synthesize blood cells, but is frequently complicated by anemia due to iron deficiency, hookworm infestation, malaria, etc.

(i) *Hepatomegaly*—The liver may be palpably enlarged. This is due to fatty infiltration of the liver which is always found post mortem in kwashiorkor.

(j) *Signs of other deficiencies*—In kwashiorkor there is usually some sub-cutaneous fat present in contrast to marasmus where there is usually none or very little. The degree of its lack gives an indication of the degree of calorie deficiency. Lesions of the lips and mouth characteristic of vitamin B deficiencies may occur. Xerosis or xerophthalmia due to vitamin A deficiency may sometimes be present.

Laboratory findings

In kwashiorkor there is usually a reduction in total serum proteins with the serum albumin content reduced more than the globulin. Serum amylase and pancreatic enzymes are also reduced as well as the ratio of essential to non-essential amino acids. Liver biopsy reveals fatty infiltration but despite the presence of edema there is no albumin in the urine.

Treatment

All severe cases should, if possible, be admitted to a hospital for treatment. Severity is judged by the amount of edema, the extent of dermatosis, the hemoglobin level, the severity of diarrhea, vomiting and dehydration, the willingness of the child to feed, but above all by the general clinical condition of the patient.

Dried skimmed milk is a most satisfactory basis for treatment, but other protein-rich foods are effective. A mixture of dried skimmed milk, vegatable oil and casein is ideal, and if necessary the child can be given the mixture through an intragastric tube. The milk mixture should provide about 120 calories and 7

Figure 4c
Supervised school lunch program in Thailand.

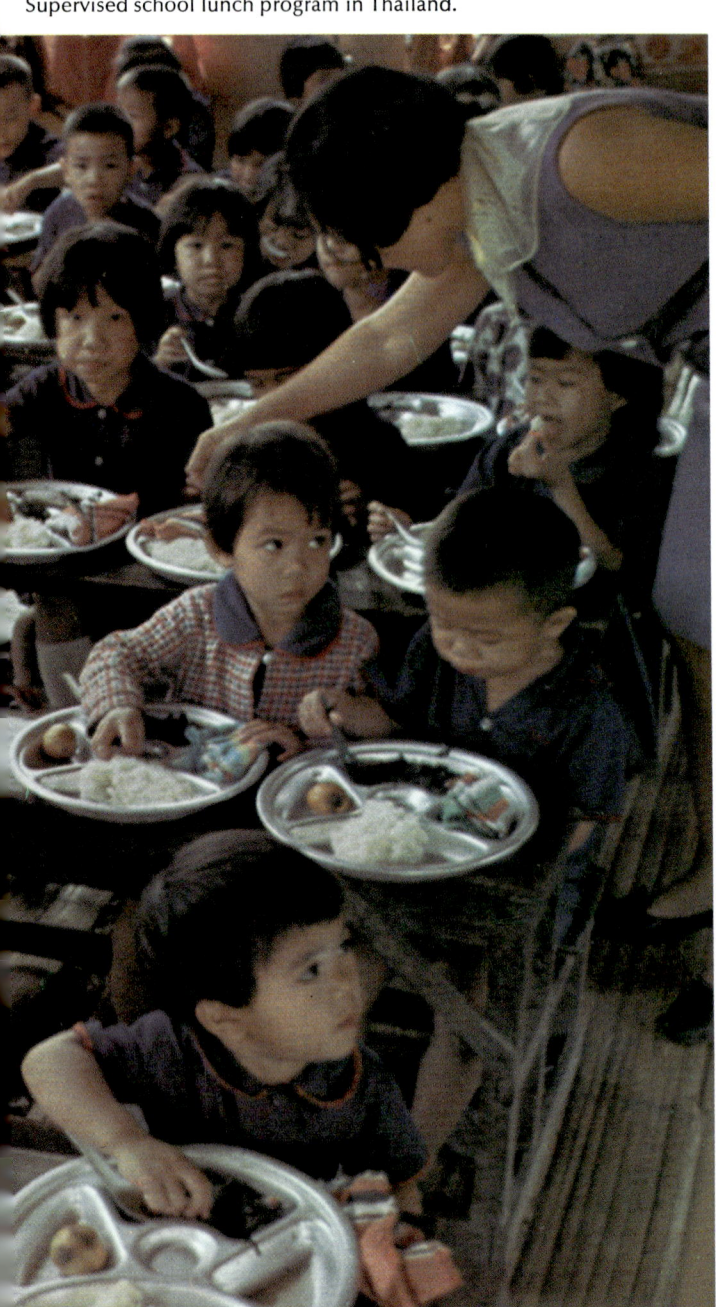

Figure 4d
School lunch in Massachusetts, U.S.A.

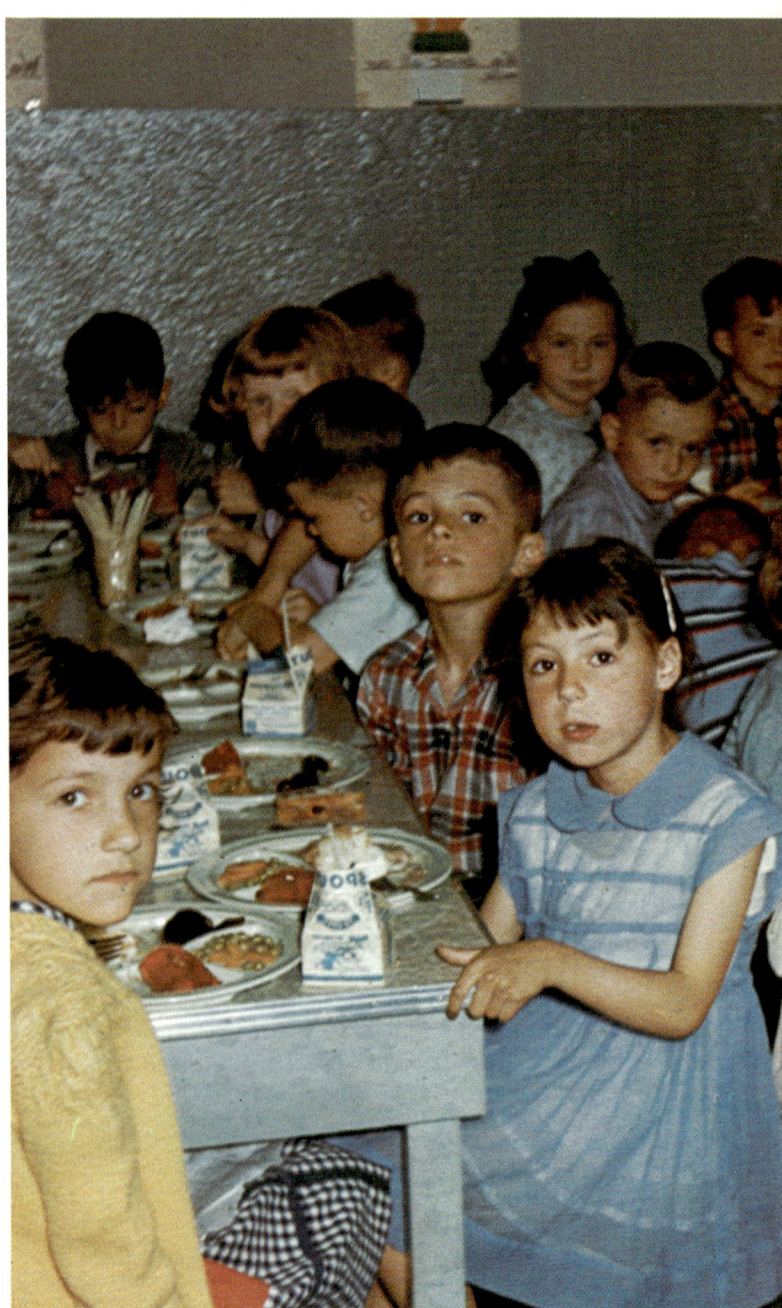

Therefore, if dried skimmed milk is used as the basis for treatment, vegetable oil should be added to provide calories.

Anemia, infections, diarrhea and dehydration should be treated as described for kwashiorkor. In general, response to treatment in severe nutritional marasmus is slow and prolonged hospitalization is often necessary.

It is particularly important to ensure that the child is not discharged from treatment back to the very set of circumstances that led to the disease. Steps must be taken to insure that an adequate diet is provided for the child after it leaves the hospital.

CLINICAL FEATURES OF KWASHIORKOR AND MARASMUS COMPARED[15]

Clinical Feature	Kwashiorkor	Marasmus
Growth Failure	Present	Present
Edema	Present	Absent
Mental Changes	Present	Uncommon
Hepatomegaly	Common	Uncommon
Hair Changes	Common	Uncommon
Dermatosis (flaky paint)	Fairly Common	Absent
Anemia	Very Common	Common
Sub-Cutaneous Fat	Reduced but Present	Absent
Appetite	Poor	Good

15. Latham, M. C., adapted from *Human Nutrition in Tropical Africa*, FAO, Rome 1966.

MILD TO MODERATE PROTEIN-CALORIE MALNUTRITION

Although detailed descriptions have been given of kwashiorkor and nutritional marasmus it should be kept in mind that these are extreme clinical conditions in the wide spectrum which constitutes protein-calorie malnutrition. In hospital practice many intermediate forms will be encountered. More important however is the fact that for every clinical case of one of these diseases there are hundreds of children who have mild or moderate forms of protein-calorie malnutrition. From a public health point of view it is desirable to try to detect these mild cases and in some way to prevent them from becoming severe.

The best means of detecting mild degrees of protein-calorie malnutrition is to follow the growth and development of young children. A child who fails to grow normally is a candidate for severe protein-calorie malnutrition and the one factor which most frequently leads to a deterioration of nutritional status is an infectious disease.

Ideally, heights, weights and other parameters of development should be followed secularly in all children at risk. If this is not possible then growth failure indicated by low height or weight for age, forms a useful guide. There are at present no biochemical tests sufficiently developed which provide a better means of detecting early protein-calorie malnutrition than the measurement of height and weight.

A grading of malnutrition on the basis of weight for age is widely used in developing countries. This is the Gomez classification:[16]

Grade I Malnutrition—75 to 90% of expected weight for age

Grade II Malnutrition—60 to 75% of expected weight for age

Grade III Malnutrition—less than 60% of expected weight for age

Weight of course, can be lost very rapidly in a sick child or from gross dietary deficiencies. In contrast height once acquired cannot be lost except in aging adulthood. Height deficits therefore, provide a better indication of chronic malnutrition. However, height expressed as a percentage of normal height gives a false picture in that it indicates smaller deficits than does weight. It is better to state height age as a percentage of actual age.[17] For example, if the standard

16. Gomez, F., *J. Trop. Pediatrics* 2:77, 1956.
17. Latham, M. C., in *Calorie Deficiencies and Protein Deficiencies*, edited by McCance and Widdowson, J. and A. Churchill Ltd., London, 1968.

Figure 6
Malnutrition may be precipitated by infection. An unsanitary environment may lead to infectious disease and parasitosis.

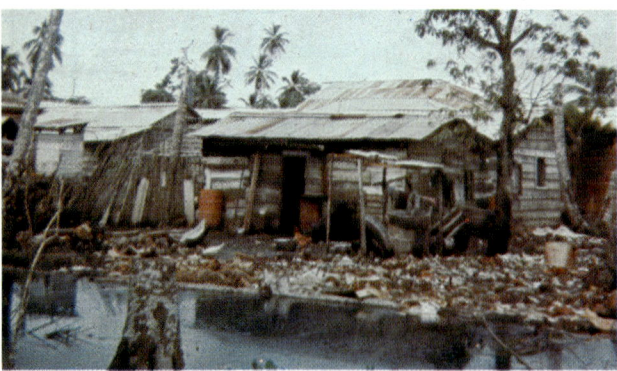

age for reaching 84 cm. in height is 24 months then a child who is 84 cm. at age 36 months is 66 per cent of his height age.

Other anthropometric measures that have practical value include head circumference, chest circumference, upper arm circumference and skinfold thickness.[18]

MALNUTRITION AND SUBSEQUENT DEVELOPMENT

There is good scientific evidence to show that children who have suffered from protein-calorie malnutrition early in life have some permanent stunting of physical growth. Therefore, if the malnutrition has been prolonged serious dwarfing may result.

There is some evidence to suggest that protein-calorie malnutrition early in life may also result in failure of the child to reach his full potential of intellectual and psychological development.[19] In experimental animals it has been shown that behavioral abnormalities follow early malnutrition. It has also been found that baby rats malnourished during the suckling period subsequently have reduced numbers of cells in the brain.[20] This has been done by relating DNA to cell numbers.

A few studies have indicated that children who have had malnutrition early in life subsequently perform less well on a variety of mental tests than do children of the same age who have not had malnutrition. There are indications that malnourished children may never catch up to the other children in intelligence.[21] Some studies have also shown that the malnourished children also have reduced head circumference, a measure which may provide an indication of brain size.[22]

18. Jelliffe, D. B., *The Assessment of the Nutritional Status of the Community*, WHO, Geneva, 1966.
19. Cravioto, J., DeLicardie, E. R., and Birch, H. G., *Pediatrics, Suppl. 38*:369, 1966.
20. Winick, M. and Noble, A., *J. Nutr. 89*:300, 1966.
21. Monckeberg, F., in *Malnutrition, Learning and Behavior*, edited by Scrimshaw and Gordon, M.I.T. Press, Cambridge, 1968.
22. Stoch, M. B. and Smythe, P. M., *South African Med. J. 41*:1027, 1967.

Research on the relationship of malnutrition to behavioral development is barely beginning. Therefore, although a definite association has been demonstrated between early protein-calorie malnutrition and subsequent poor intellectual performance it has not been proved that this relationship is one of cause and effect. Quite possibly some genetic and environmental factors which influence intellectual development of children may also be important in the etiology of malnutrition. Therefore, factors such as poverty, ignorant and illiterate parents, crowding, a high prevalence of infectious disease, poor learning opportunities and several others may be causes both of malnutrition and of poor psychological development in children.

NUTRITION AND INFECTION

In recent years the importance of the synergism of infection and dietary deficiencies in the causation of severe protein-calorie malnutrition has been realized.[23,24] The corollary is equally true, namely, that malnutrition is largely responsible for the increased severity and many of the devastating effects of infectious disease in malnourished children. Gastroenteritis, measles and other infections may frequently precipitate clinical malnutrition in a child. Similarly, diseases like measles which have a very low mortality in the well-nourished often have a high mortality in populations where malnutrition is prevalent.

Diarrheal disease in children at an age when they are being weaned from the breast is extremely common in developing countries and has been termed "weanling diarrhea." This is now commonly known to be a precipitating cause of malnutrition. It is also now clear that malnourished children more frequently develop diarrhea than do the well-nourished and that frequently the diarrhea may be due to malnutrition and not a pathogenic organism.

23. *Nutrition and Infection*, World Health Organization Technical Reports Series No. 314, WHO, Geneva, 1965.
24. Scrimshaw, N. S., Taylor, C. E., and Gordon, J. E., *Am. J. Med. Sci. 237*:367, 1959.

Xerophthalmia-Keratomalacia

Keratomalacia is a disease which is almost unknown in the United States, but is a common cause of blindness in some parts of the world, particularly in certain countries of Asia and the Middle East.[25] It is due to a dietary deficiency of vitamin A and occurs in young children and is often associated with protein-calorie malnutrition.

The Disease

An early sign of vitamin A deficiency is night blindness or the inability to see well in dim light. This is difficult to detect in young children. Vitamin A deficiency may also cause follicular hyperkeratosis of the skin and Bitot's spots of the eyes.

Xerophthalmia usually begins with a drying of the conjunctiva which loses its shining luster. This condition may then spread to the cornea which also becomes dull and loses its power to reflect. This pathological dryness of the eye, which robs it of its normal epithelial protection, is called xerophthalmia and is a precursor of keratomalacia.

If the condition remains untreated a necrotic process begins, followed by ulceration and leads to perforation, loss of intraocular fluid and a severe secondary infection may occur. The patient at this stage is often seriously ill with pyrexia and a grossly inflamed eye, and the patient is doomed to blindness in the afflicted eye.

If treatment is begun early or if food rich in vitamin A is consumed before the stage of perforation, then the ulcer may heal leaving perhaps only an opaque corneal scar. In some cases vascularization of the cornea precedes ulceration.

In vitamin A deficiency the concentration of vitamin A in the plasma is usually below 20 μg. per 100 ml. but may be so low as to be undetectable and it must be low for a prolonged period to produce clinical signs of vitamin A deficiency. Normal levels range from 30 to 50 μg. per 100 ml.

25. Oomen, H. A., McLaren, D. S., and Escapini, U., *Trop. Geograph. Med.* 16:271, 1964.

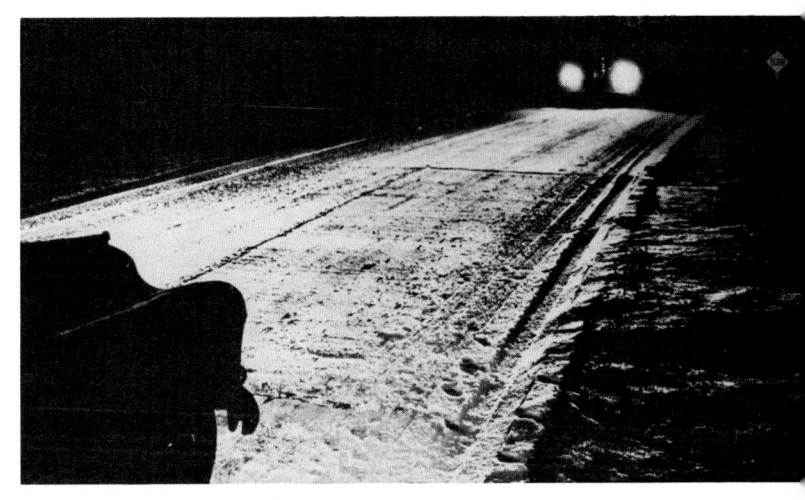

Figure 7a
Vitamin A Deficiency—Night Blindness is a useful and early diagnostic sign of vitamin A deficiency. The loss of visual acuity in dim light following exposure to bright light is illustrated.

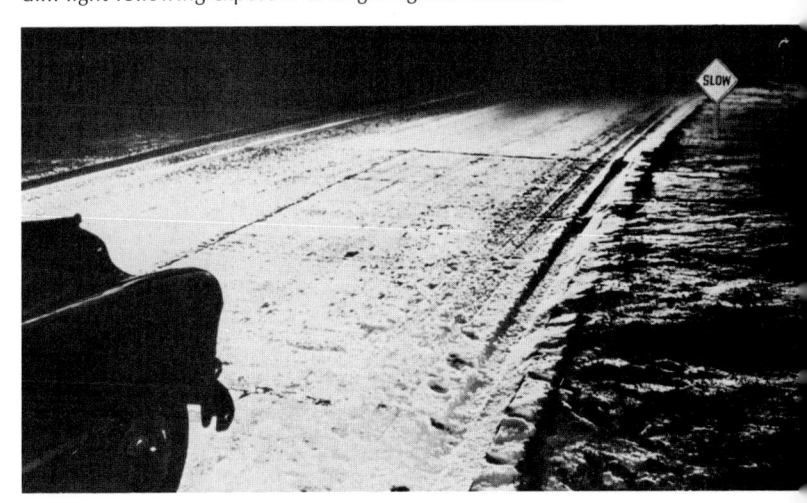

Figure 7b
Both the normal individual and the vitamin A deficient subject see the headlights of an approaching car as shown in *Figure 7b*. After the car has passed the normal individual sees a wide stretch of road.

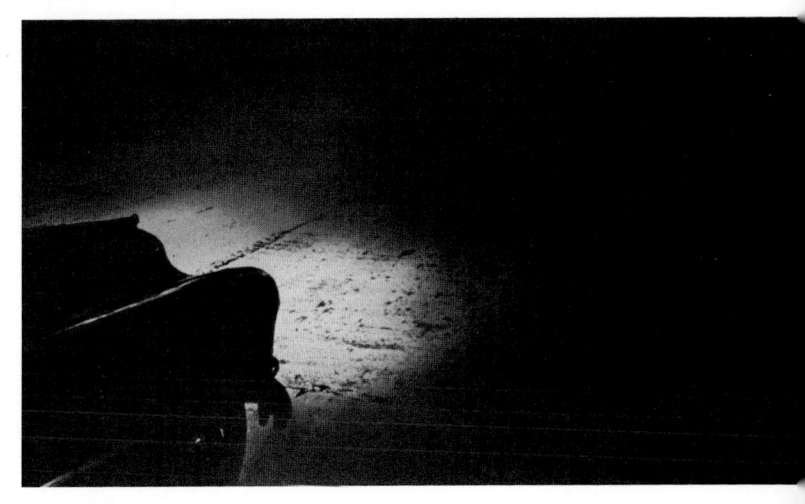

Figure 7c
The vitamin A-deficient subject can barely see a few feet ahead and cannot see the road sign at all.

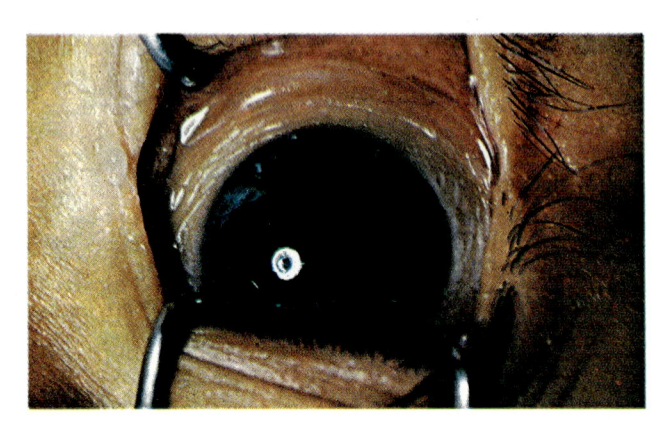

Figure 8
Bitots spots—white foamy plaques on the temporal side of the cornea.

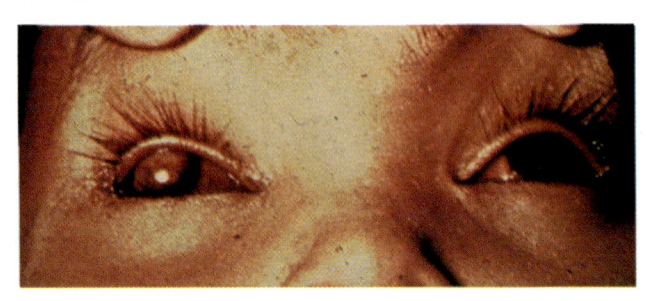

Figure 9
Xerophthalmia in an Indonesian child with severe involvement of one eye.

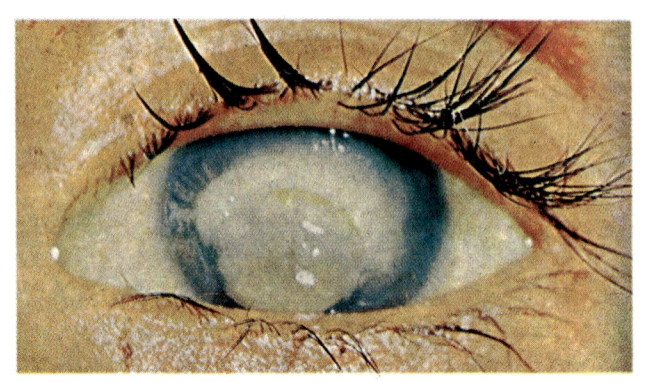

Figure 10
Keratomalacia in a young child.

Treatment
Severe cases of xerophthalmia should be treated as a medical emergency as the sight and life of the children is at stake. The recommended treatment is:

(a) Injection of a vitamin A preparation at an initial dose of 22.5 mg. (75,000 I.U.)

(b) 22.5 mg. (75,000 I.U.) vitamin A daily by mouth. This may be either a preparation of synthetic vitamin A or in the form of cod- or halibut-liver oil.

(c) Tetracycline or other antibiotic eye ointments should be instilled into both eyes every four hours for the first 48 hours and less frequently for the next 7 to 10 days.

(d) Riboflavin tablets 5 mg. three times daily.

(e) For a period of 7 to 10 days penicillin 600,000 units daily I.M. or some other antibiotic should be administered to combat secondary infection.

(f) A mixed diet, rich in vitamin A and carotene should be given.

(g) Protein-calorie malnutrition should be treated if present.

Thiamine Deficiency Syndromes Including Beriberi and the Wernicke-Korsakoff Syndrome

Beriberi
Beriberi is caused by a deficiency of the B vitamin thiamine, also known as B_1, when the ratio of its intake to the number of calories obtained from carbohydrate is low. The disease occurs predominantly among rice-eating peoples of the world because of the desire for refined or polished rice.

The Disease
There are various ways of dividing beriberi from a clinical viewpoint. Here it will be grouped into three forms: (1) Wet beriberi, (2) Dry beriberi, and (3) Infantile beriberi. These three clinical forms of the

disease have many different features and yet appear to be caused by the same dietary deficiency and occur in the same endemic areas.

Early clinical features common to both wet and dry beriberi

Both wet and dry beriberi usually begin in a similar mild way. The person tires easily, his limbs feel heavy and weak and he may get a mild degree of swelling around the ankles. There may be a numbness and a feeling of "pins and needles" in the legs, as well as occasional palpitations of the heart.

Examination at this stage might reveal some reduced motor power, perhaps a slight alteration in gait and a patchy anesthesia over the skin of the lower legs. The rice eater in the orient or the alcoholic elsewhere will often continue his normal activities and not seek early medical advice. The condition at this stage would improve with a better diet or with thiamine administration. Left untreated, the condition might remain almost static for months but at any stage might progress to either clinical wet or dry beriberi.

Wet beriberi

The name wet beriberi is used because the main feature of the disease is the accumulation of edema fluid in the legs and often in the scrotum, face and trunk. The patient frequently develops cardiac palpitations, chest pain and later dyspnea. The pulse is rapid and often irregular. The neck veins are distended with visible pulsations and the heart becomes enlarged. The volume of urine tends to be diminished but despite the edema contains no albumin. This latter is an important diagnostic feature.

A patient with wet beriberi is in danger of rapid deterioration, acute circulatory failure, and death.

Dry beriberi

This is termed dry because edema is not a feature. The condition is really neuritic beriberi and is similar to peripheral neuritis due to other causes.

Anesthesia and paresthesia of the feet followed by increased difficulty in walking is a common feature. On examination the patient has a peculiar ataxic gait, foot drop and wrist drop are common, there is considerable muscular wasting, there are anesthetic patches especially over the tibia and there is tenderness of the calves and other muscles when pressure is applied. The sufferer has great difficulty in rising from the squatting position.

The disease is often chronic, and at any stage improvement may slowly occur if the subject consumes a better diet or receives treatment with thiamine. Untreated the disease progresses, the patient eventually becomes bed ridden and frequently dies of some chronic infection.

Infantile beriberi

This is the only important dietary deficiency disease which occurs in otherwise normal infants under six months of age who are receiving adequate quantities of breast milk. It is due to inadequate thiamine in the milk of a lactating mother whose diet is deficient in this vitamin. The mother may however, have no overt signs of beriberi.

Infantile beriberi commonly occurs between 2 and 6 months of age. In the acute form the infant develops dyspnea and cyanosis and dies of cardiac failure with unnerving rapidity. In chronic forms, the classical sign is aphonia, the infant going through the motions of crying like a well rehearsed mime, but without emitting much of any sound. The infant is thin and wasted, diarrhea and vomiting may develop and due to a deficiency of calories and other nutrients the infant becomes marasmic. Edema occasionally is seen and convulsions may occur in the terminal stages.

Diagnosis of wet, dry and infantile beriberi

Diagnosis may be difficult when only the early manifestations are present. A history of a diet deficient in thiamine and improvement on a good diet or following treatment with thiamine will help to establish the diagnosis.

Wet beriberi must be distinguished from renal edema and congestive cardiac failure. In both these latter conditions there is albuminuria; in beriberi there is not.

Measurement of blood levels of thiamine and thiamine phosphate is of limited value. More useful are determinations of blood lactate and blood pyruvate levels especially if performed after glucose administration and exercise. Urinary excretion of thiamine per gram of creatinine provides a good index of thiamine intake but is useful for surveys rather than for diagnosis in the individual patient.

Treatment

Wet beriberi

(a) Absolute bed rest.

(b) Thiamine 10 to 20 mg. daily by injection. When clinical improvement is evident replace injections with oral thiamine 10 mg. daily.

(c) Full nutritious diet rich in B vitamins but low in carbohydrate.

Severe wet beriberi is a very gratifying disease to treat for the response is usually dramatic. Diuresis and rapid reduction of dyspnea occur with elimination of edema in a few days.

Dry beriberi

(a) Rest in bed.

(b) Thiamine 10 mg. daily by mouth.

(c) Nutritious diet including B complex vitamins.

(d) Physiotherapy.

Improvement is often very slow.

Infantile beriberi

(a) Immediate injection of thiamine 5 mg. and daily injections for four days.

(b) Thiamine 10 mg. orally twice a day to the mother if the child is being breast fed.

(c) Nutritious and thiamine-rich diet to both mother and child.

Thiamine deficiency in the U.S.

Although classical beriberi is uncommon in the U.S., thiamine deficiency is by no means a rarity. It is

Figure 11
Edema in beriberi.

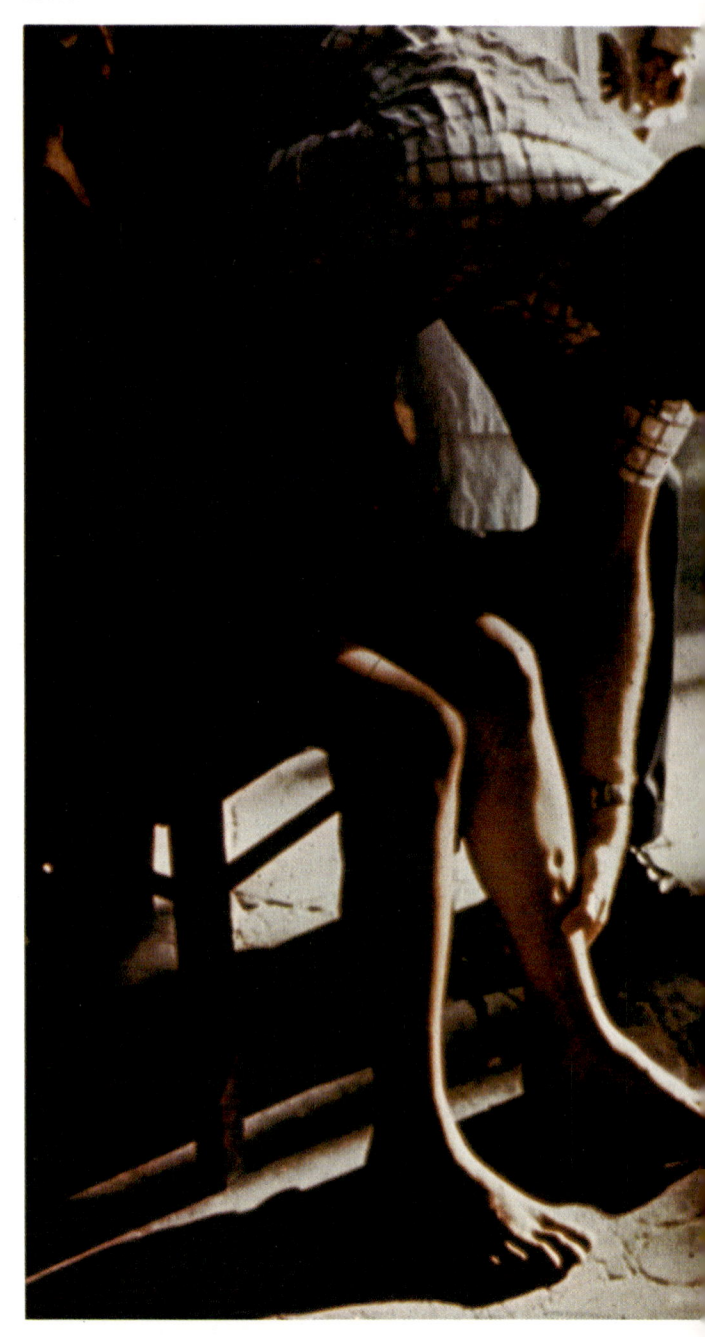

confined mainly to the alcoholic population. Alcoholism is an increasingly prevalent condition and several clinical features previously believed to be due to chronic alcoholic intoxication are now known to be the result of nutritional deficiencies.

Wernicke-Korsakoff Syndrome

Wernicke's disease is characterized by eye signs (nystagmus, diplopia, paralysis of the externi recti muscles and sometimes ophthalmoplegia), ataxia and mental changes. Korsakoff's psychosis leads to a loss of memory of the immediate past and often an elaborate confabulation which tends to conceal this amnesia.

It is now generally agreed that any distinction between Wernicke's disease and Korsakoff's psychosis may be artificial in the alcoholic patient. Korsakoff's psychosis may be regarded as the psychotic component of Wernicke's disease.[26]

This view is supported by the fact that many patients who appear with ocular palsy, ataxia and confusion and who survive, later show the amnestic disorder of Korsakoff's psychosis. Similarly patients in mental institutions with Korsakoff's psychosis often show the stigmata of Wernicke's disease even years after the illness. Pathological evidence also indicates the unity of the two conditions.

Proof that the Wernicke-Korsakoff syndrome is due to thiamine deficiency and not to chronic alcohol intoxication is shown by the fact that the condition responds to thiamine alone, even if the individual continues to consume alcohol.

Of overriding importance in this syndrome is the fact that irreversible brain damage ensues rapidly and therefore early recognition and treatment are vital. If there is any suspicion that a patient may have this condition, he should immediately receive 5 to 10 mg. of thiamine by injection even before a definitive diagnosis is made.

Prevention

The prevention of the Wernicke-Korsakoff syndrome calls for considerable public health ingenuity. Possibilities suggested[27] have included:

(a) The "immunization" of alcoholics with large doses of thiamine at regular intervals. The development of a suitable depot carrier to reduce the frequency of these injections would be very helpful.

(b) The fortification of alcoholic beverages with thiamine.

(c) A provision by public health authorities that thiamine impregnated snacks be available on bar counters.

The cost of any of these measures would almost certainly be less than is the present enormous expenditure on institutional care of those who have suffered from Wernicke-Korsakoff disease.

Other thiamine deficiency states

Alcoholic polyneuropathy, a condition similar to neuritic beriberi, is also a disease due to a dietary deficiency of thiamine.

An optic or retrobulbar neuritis which occurred in prison camps in World War II was probably due to thiamine deficiency. This condition, also known as nutritional amblyopia was at least in part due to thiamine deficiency.

Pellagra

Pellagra which used to be common in the southern United States is now seldom seen in this country. The disease is associated with a corn (maize) diet and is primarily due to a dietary deficiency of niacin. Although corn has more niacin than some other staple foods it seems that this is not all utilized, most likely because it is in a bound form unavailable to the body. The human body can convert the amino acid tryptophan into niacin and so a high-protein diet rich in tryptophan will help prevent pellagra. The main protein in corn is zein which is very low in tryptophan content.

26. Victor, M. and Adams, R. D., *Am. J. Clin. Nutr.* 9:379, 1961.

27. Latham, M. C., in *Present Knowledge in Nutrition*, The Nutrition Foundation, Inc., New York 1967.

The Disease

Pellagra to the medical student is portrayed by the four D's– dermatitis, diarrhea, dementia, and death. The disease is most often diagnosed from the characteristic appearance of the skin lesions. These lesions are often symmetrical in appearance and occur on areas of the body exposed to sunlight such as the face, the neck and the forearms. In Caucasians the skin lesions at first resemble the erythema of sunburn. In Negroes there is a hyperpigmentation. The affected areas become dry, scaly and cracked and if the condition progresses desquamation commonly occurs. There may be cracking and fissuring, and occasionally the skin becomes blistered. In persons wearing an open-neck shirt, the upper chest and lower neck are affected and this lesion is known as Casal's neckline.

Digestive symptoms include abdominal pain and diarrhea. Frequently the tongue and mouth are sore, and sometimes angular stomatitis and cheilosis, usually associated with riboflavin deficiency, occur. The tongue is often red, smooth and raw looking.

Involvement of the nervous system manifests itself by extremely variable symptoms and signs. The commonest of these are irritability, loss of memory, insomnia and anxiety. These may lead to dementia. It used to be common for persons to be incarcerated in mental institutions without anyone realizing that the mental condition was due to pellagra. In areas where corn is the primary staple food all persons admitted to mental institutions should be examined for evidence of pellagra.

Mild sensory and motor changes occasionally occur in pellagra, but paralysis is very rare.

Diagnosis

Diagnosis is usually made on the basis of the dietary history and on physical examination.

Treatment

Hospital admission is only necessary for very serious cases. Niacinamide 50 to 100 mg. three times daily by intramuscular injection for the first 3-4 days

Figure 12a
Casal's Necklace—Advanced Pellagra. Dermatitis outlining the exposed area of the neck is pathognomonic of pellagra, as are the characteristic lesions on the backs of the hands. Either sunlight or heat from a stove may have been the precipitating factor.

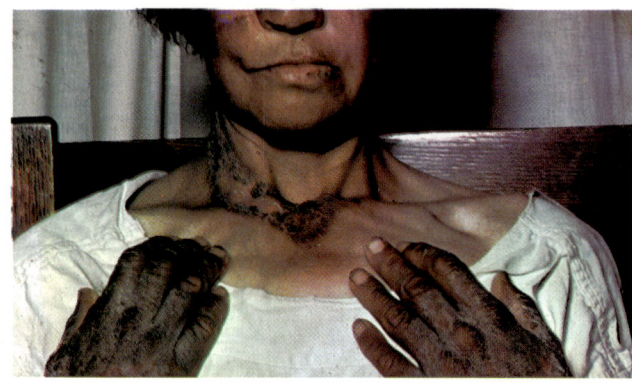

Figure 12b
Same patient after nicotinamide therapy.

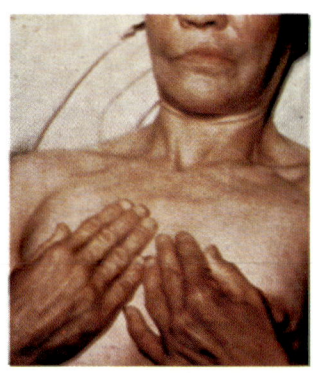

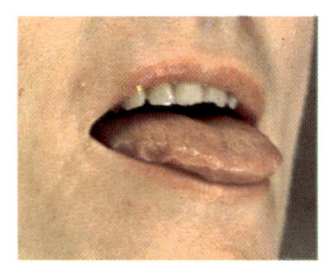

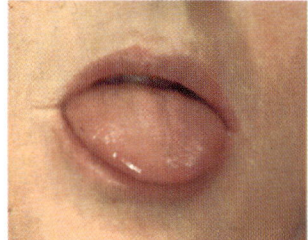

Figure 13a   *Figure 13b*

Glossitis is the earliest diagnostic sign of pellagra brought about by nicotinamide deficiency. It starts with a burning sensation, which is followed either by edema or by desquamation of the epithelium. Dental indentations *(Figure 13a)* result from edema. Tip and margins of tongue are made scarlet red and shiny by desquamation of the epithelium *(Figure 13b)*. There are signs of healed angular stomatitis, indicating a previous riboflavin deficiency.

and subsequently by mouth should form the basis of treatment. A daily diet of high caloric value and containing at least 100 grams of good quality protein is recommended.

If abdominal burning or diarrhea are troublesome, an easily digestable diet low in fiber content should be given. Sedation with barbiturates is recommended for the first few days of treatment. Those with mental disturbances benefit greatly from a tranquilizer prescribed in relatively large doses. A vitamin B complex preparation is useful to counteract concurrent deficiencies of other B vitamins.

Scurvy

Today scurvy is a rare disease. It results from a deficiency of vitamin C and usually occurs only after a considerable time in persons on a diet containing very little fresh food. Daily intakes of vitamin C very much below the recommended allowances, even for periods of several months, usually do not result in scurvy.

Vitamin C is necessary for the formation and healthy upkeep of intercellular material. In scurvy the walls of the capillaries lack solidity and become fragile resulting in hemorrhage from various sites.

The Disease

The following symptoms and signs may occur:

(a) Tenderness of the extremities, muscle weakness and suppressed appetite.

(b) Gums become swollen and bleed easily; teeth may become loose.

(c) Hemorrhages of a petechial type often occur in the skin.

(d) Hemorrhages in other areas may manifest themselves as nose bleeds, hematuria, melena, splinter hemorrhages below the nails and painful sub-periosteal hemorrhages.

(e) Delayed healing of wounds and heightened risk of infection.

(f) Anemia and shortness of breath.

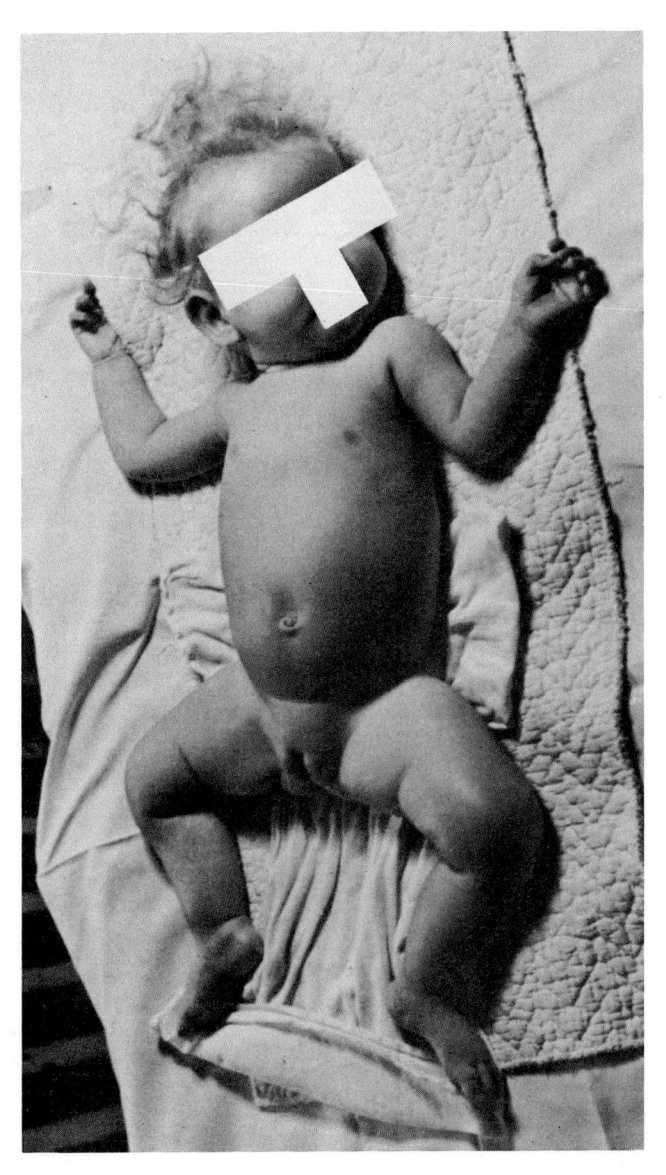

Figure 14
Infant with scurvy in the "Pithed Frog" position. Because movement is painful, the scorbutic infant usually lies on its back and makes little attempt to lift the leg or arm that hurts. Both legs may be tender, and sometimes both arms as well. This is usually the first sign of scurvy.

A patient with scurvy and some of the above symptoms and signs, though not appearing very seriously ill, may suddenly collapse and die of cardiac failure.

Infantile scurvy (Barlow's disease)

Infantile scurvy usually occurs in infants, 2 to 12 months of age, who are bottle fed with a milk formula to which vitamin C has not been added and who do not receive any other source of vitamin C. The vitamin C in milk is destroyed by heat in the pasteurization or drying of milk.

The infant with scurvy cries when the limbs are touched or moved due to pain and tenderness. The infant often lies with his limbs placed in what has been called the "pithed frog" position. Swellings due to hemorrhages may be felt especially in the legs and there may be obvious bruising of the body. Hemorrhages may occur from any of the sites mentioned previously for adult scurvy but gum bleeding does not occur unless there are erupted teeth.

Diagnosis of Scurvy

The capillary fragility test is useful but there are other conditions beside scurvy which influence capillary strength. Estimations of ascorbic acid in serum, or preferably in white blood cells, may be useful. If serum ascorbic acid is present, the disease is not scurvy. Decreased urinary excretion of ascorbic acid is an early sign. Radiographs aid in the diagnosis of infantile scurvy and in older subjects "scurvy lines" of the tibia and femur are helpful in the diagnosis.

The concentration of ascorbic acid in the blood plasma reflects the dietary intake and does not indicate the degree of depletion of the bodily stores. It is better to measure the concentration of ascorbic acid in the leukocytes. Levels below 2 mg./100 ml. provide presumptive evidence of scurvy.

Treatment

Because of the danger of sudden death, even in the patient who looks reasonably well, there is a need for immediate vigorous treatment. It is advisable to give by mouth a loading dose of 1000 mg. ascorbic acid followed by 250 mg. four times daily for 6 to 7 days when the dosage can usually be reduced to 50 mg. twice a day until recovery is complete. The patient should also be put on a diet containing plenty of fresh fruit and vegetables. Ascorbic acid by injection is necessary if the patient is vomiting and is useful for the treatment of infants.

Rickets and Osteomalacia

In both rickets and osteomalacia there is a lack of calcium retention in the skeleton. The conditions are, however, due mainly to a deficiency of vitamin D and not of dietary calcium. Vitamin D is obtained both from the diet and from exposure of the skin to sunlight. The average unsupplemented diet contains only relatively small amounts of vitamin D but nowadays this vitamin is added to many processed foods, especially those commonly consumed by young children. Vitamin D deficiency is therefore uncommon in children and is very rare in adults in the United States.

RICKETS

The Disease

Unlike many other deficiency diseases the child with rickets often has the superficial appearance of being plump and well fed. This frequently gives the mother a false sense of security. The story has often been told of the rachitic child winning the baby show because it appeared so fat and well nourished. The child, however, tends to be miserable and closer examination will reveal the flabby toneless state of the muscles. Another feature is the general impairment of normal development. The child is frequently late in reaching all the milestones in his early life. He is slow to learn to sit, to walk and to get his teeth. Other generalized signs include gastrointestinal upsets and excessive sweating of the head.

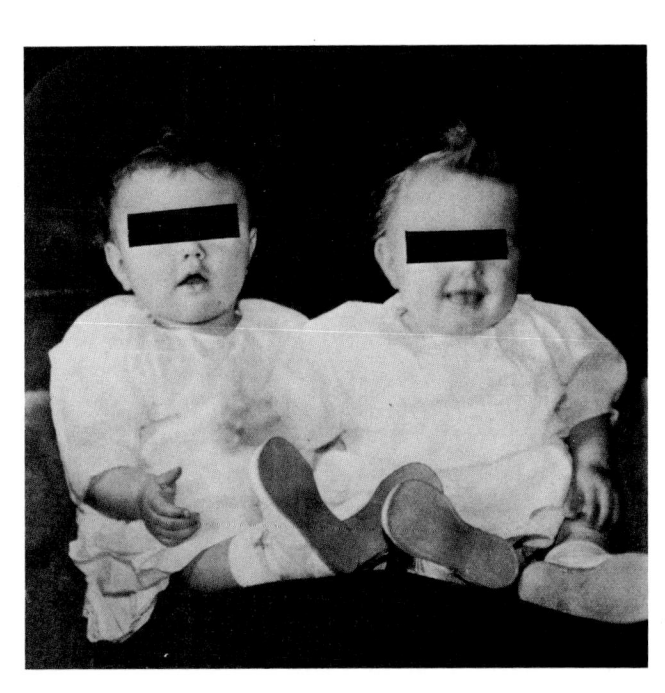

Figure 15
Two Girls with Rickets: The cases of Ethel and Evelyn
These patients, twins, were first seen on July 10, two days after they had won first prize at a baby show. Both infants were female and appeared to be well nourished. They were markedly obese. On physical examination, there was a definite craniotabes. The anterior fontanelle was open. There was a flaring of the lower rib margin and a well marked rachitic rosary. There was an extreme bowing of both legs, which was more marked in the lower third. "X-ray films of the legs and ankles showed a marked flaring and widening of the diaphesis above the epiphyseal line. The zone between the shaft and the epihysis is increased in thickness with ragged, fringy margins. There is a marked bowing of the lower end of the tibia."   Diagnosis–Rachitis-Infant

These children had been raised on artificial feeding with no supplemental vitamin D. They were placed on high doses of vitamin D concentrate. A very rapid improvement was noted in both cases, especially that of Ethel, whose condition was so severe that she was placed in bed with traction on both feet. We were not able to secure X-ray films again until February 7. At this time there was an increase in the density of the bone with a marked thickening of the cortex of the shaft on the concave side. The epiphyseal line is much narrower and the margin is much more regular in outline.

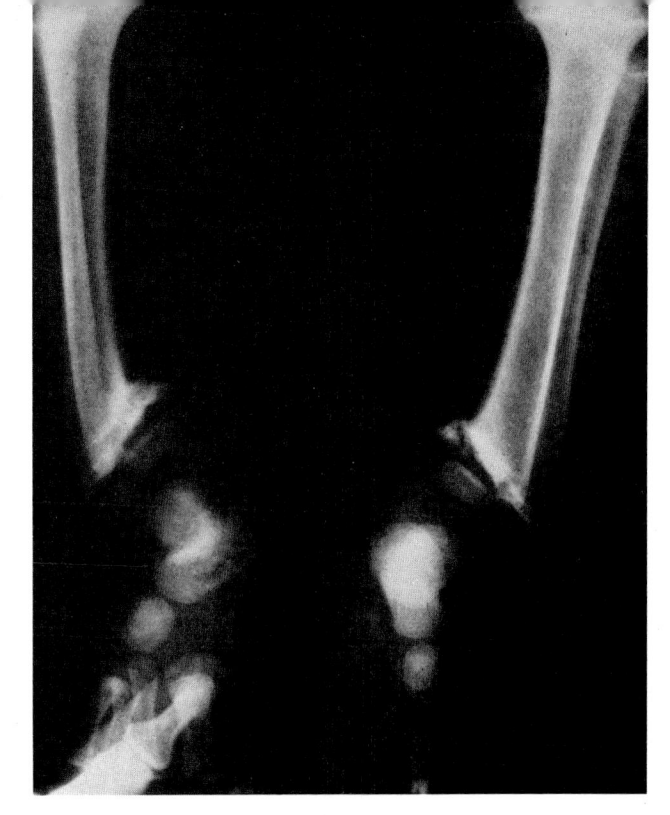

Figure 16a
7-10-35, Roentgenologic Findings (Right and Left Legs and Ankles). X-ray films of the legs and ankles show a marked flaring and widening of the diaphysis above the epiphyseal line. The zone between the shaft and epiphysis is increased in thickness with ragged fringy margins. There is a marked bowing of the lower end of tibia.   Conclusion–Rachitic infant

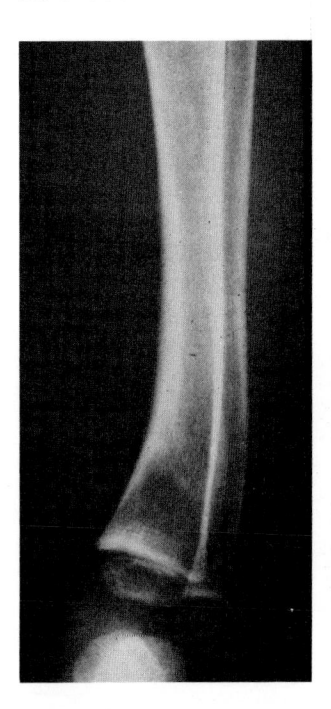

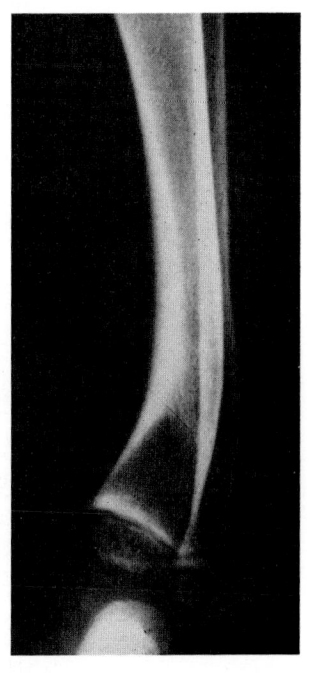

Figure 16b
2-7-36, Roentgenologic Findings (Right and Left Legs and Ankles). X-ray films after treatment show an increase in the density of the bone. There is a marked thickening of the cortex of the shaft on the concave side. The epiphyseal line is much narrower and the margin is much more regular in outline.
   Conclusion–X-ray films show a marked improvement.

Figure 17a
Child from moderately well-to-do family with marked bow legs due to rickets.

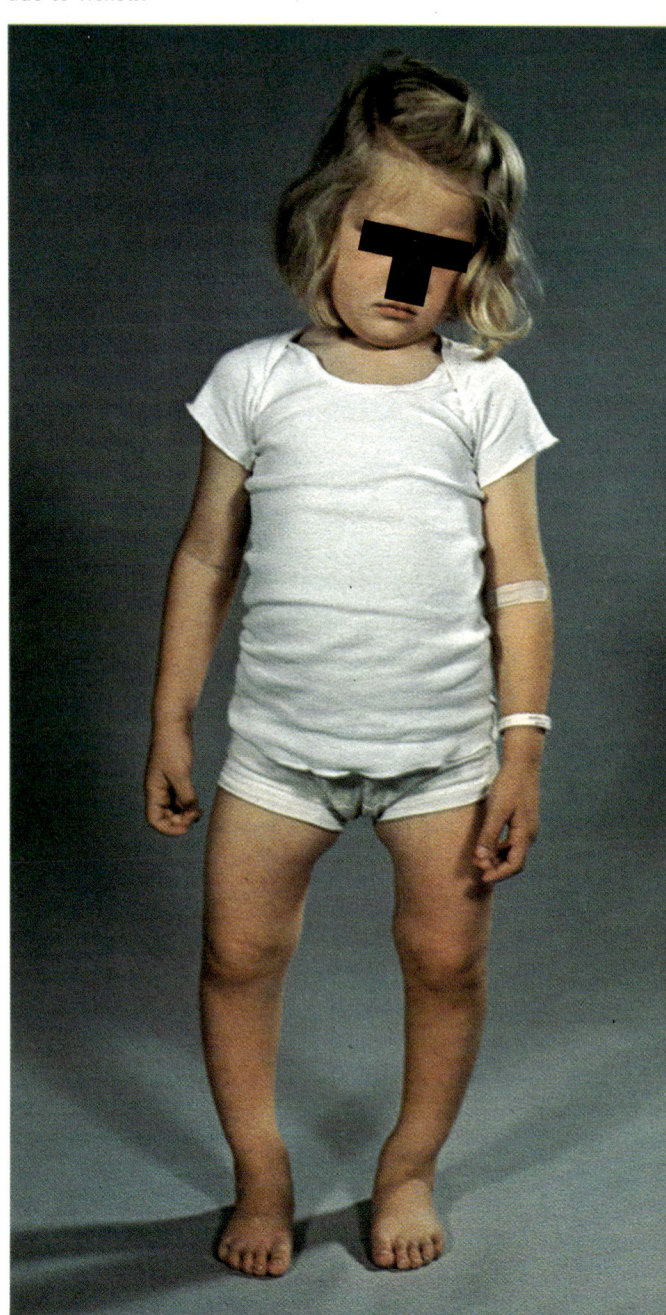

The main signs of the disease and those on which the diagnosis of rickets is made are the skeletal changes. One early feature is a swelling of the epiphysis of the long bones. This may first be found at the wrist where the radius is affected. Another classical site is at the costo-chondral junctions where swellings occur. This produces a bead-like appearance which has received the name "rachitic rosary." Deformities of the chest lead to the formation of Harrison's sulcus and pigeon breast. Swellings of the epiphyses of the tibia, fibula and femur may also be seen.

In young infants craniotabes is often the first sign of rickets. This consists of areas of softening of the skull usually affecting the occipital and parietal bones. There is also delayed closing of the anterior fontanel. In severe rickets there may be bossing of the skull.

When a child with rickets begins to stand and walk he often develops new deformities due to the soft, weak character of the bones. The commonest of these are bowlegs and less frequently knock-knees. More serious, however, are deformities of the spine leading to kyphosis. Changes in the pelvis though often not obvious may subsequently result in difficulty in childbirth in women who have had rickets during childhood.

Tetany due to a reduction in the level of serum calcium sometimes occurs. It presents an unmistakable picture with spasm of the hands; the thumb being drawn into the palm.

Diagnosis

X-ray examination will reveal abnormalities and is also helpful in showing progress during treatment. Radiographs, especially of the wrists but also of the ends of long bones at other sites are useful in diagnosis. This will usually reveal characteristic changes in the epiphyses. The outline of the joint is blurred, the epiphyseal line is broadened and later the end of the bone shaft appears saucered. The trabeculation of

Figure 19
Drawing of types of goiter.

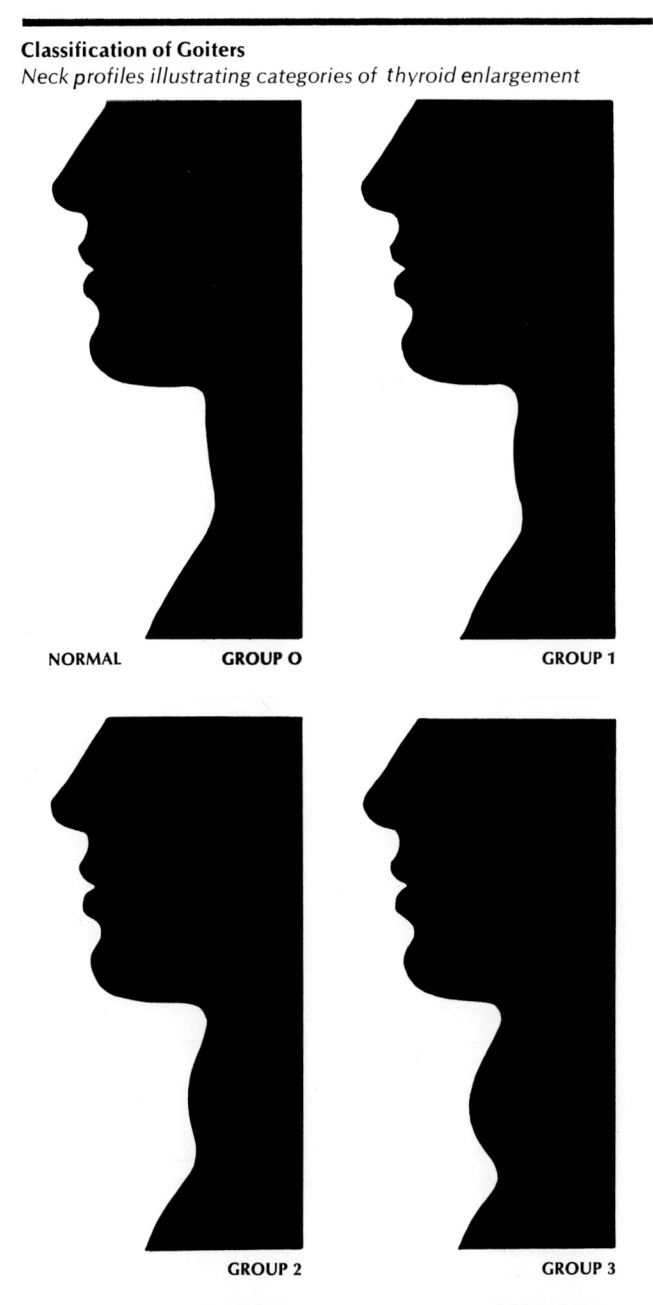

Classification of Goiters
Neck profiles illustrating categories of thyroid enlargement

NORMAL   GROUP 0   GROUP 1
GROUP 2   GROUP 3

the gland may be smooth and is then said to be a colloid goiter or it may be lumpy and is then called an adenomatous or nodular goiter.

Endemic goiter, in which there is a benign enlargement of the thyroid gland, may cause no symptoms. The enlargement is merely evidence of a deficient intake of iodine. Appropriate treatment will prevent both further enlargement and the complications which may accompany goiter and in many cases will cause the gland to return to its normal size. Untreated, the gland may enlarge to a size which is obvious and presents a cosmetic problem. Further enlargement may produce pressure symptoms such as difficulty in breathing, persistent cough or voice changes. A person with a simple goiter may develop the symptoms and signs of hyperthyroidism. Carcinoma of the thyroid is more common in those with goiter.

Cretinism in children occurs most commonly in endemic goiter areas and is almost certainly due to severe iodine deficiency of the mother. The infant might appear normal at birth, but is slow to develop, small in size, mentally dull, has a thick skin and a characteristic face with depressed nose and often a protruding, enlarged tongue. Deaf mutism and mental retardation are found more frequently in the children of mothers with enlarged thyroid glands.

Treatment

Small diffuse colloid goiters will reduce in size and may disappear with suitable iodine therapy or with an increased dietary intake of iodine. The recommended treatment is Lugol's solution of iodine 0.5 ml. per day by mouth in water.

More dramatic improvement, especially in those with larger goiters, can be achieved by the use of thyroid extract or thyroxine. If this form of therapy is used, the weight, pulse rate and if possible the basal metabolic rate of the patient should be checked at regular intervals. Treatment should start with a small dose; e.g., thyroid extract ½ gr. daily and be in-

Sea foods such as fish, shellfish and seaweed are rich sources of iodine. Endemic goiter areas are usually far from the sea.

It has been found in experimental animals that there are certain foods which if eaten in large quantities, make the animal more liable to develop goiter even if normal quantities of iodine are consumed. Substances which have this effect are called goitrogens and are known to exist in certain varieties of cabbage, kale, turnips and some other vegetables. There is little evidence to incriminate dietary goitrogens as being important in endemic goiter in man.

In the U.S.A. endemic areas of goiter are mainly in the states bordering on Canada, especially the Great Lakes area and those between the Rocky Mountains and the Appalachians.

Physiology of endemic goiter

The thyroid gland requires iodine to produce thyroxine which contains 64 per cent iodine. When iodine is deficient the gland enlarges to try to compensate for this difficulty in producing thyroxine. This basically is the mechanism at work in goiter due to iodine deficiency.

The normal thyroid gland contains about 8 milligrams of iodine and this may be reduced to 1 to 2 milligrams in persons with goiter. The thyroid gland is under the control of the anterior pituitary gland. Iodine is absorbed from the intestines at a rate which is dependent on thyroid activity. The rate of secretion of thyroid stimulating hormone (T.S.H.) by the anterior pituitary depends upon the concentration of thyroid hormones circulating in the blood. Thyroxine administration will therefore inhibit T.S.H. secretion.

The iodine uptake in normal persons is proportional to the blood concentration of the thyroid hormones. It has been shown that the uptake of radioactive iodine is increased in hyperthyroidism and decreased in hypothyroidism. There are, however, other factors which can influence it.

The total iodine content in whole blood is usually 10 μg. $\pm$ 4 μg. of which 6 μg. $\pm$ 2 μg. is protein-bound. The protein-bound iodine (PBI) is reduced in hypothyroidism and elevated in hyperthyroidism. The amount of iodine in the urine is dependent mainly on the iodine intake in the diet and on thyroid activity.

Endemic goiter is diagnosed when there is thyroid enlargement in a patient living in an area where endemic goiter is known to occur, where there is evidence that the iodine intake of the patient is low and where other causes of thyroid enlargement can be ruled out.

Urinary excretion of iodine in these individuals would usually be below 100 μg. daily, the protein-bound iodine is in the normal range and the uptake of radioactive I^{131} is often increased.

Goiter surveys

When investigating goiter prevalence in a population the thyroid gland of a representative sample should be examined both visually and by palpation in order to estimate the degree of enlargement. Each lobe of the normal thyroid gland is about the size of the thumb nail of the person being examined. A useful classification of goiter size is that suggested by W.H.O.[28] which can be summarized as follows:

Group 0–Persons without goiter and persons with the thyroid less than five times enlarged.

Group 1–Persons with the thyroid more than five times enlarged but not easily visible with the head in normal position.

Group 2–Persons with goiters which are easily visible with the head in normal position, but which are smaller than Group 3.

Group 3–Persons with large goiters which can be easily recognized at a considerable distance and which may be disfiguring.

The Disease

Goiter is more common in females particularly at puberty and during pregnancy. The enlargement of

28. *Endemic Goiter*, World Health Organization Monograph Series No. 4, WHO, Geneva, 1960.

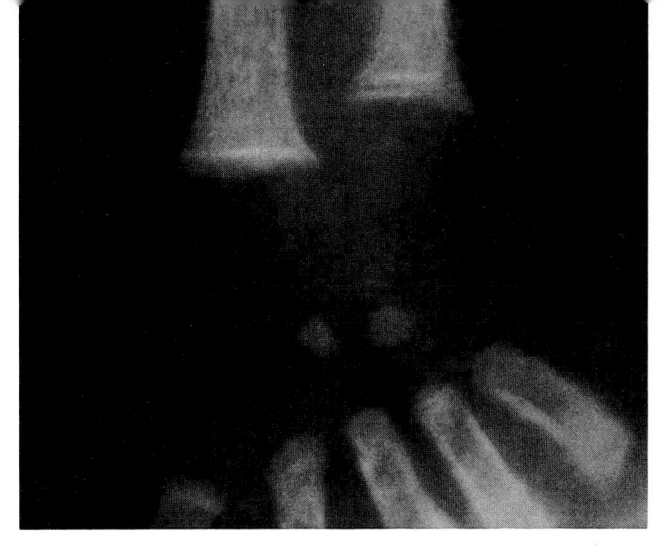

Figure 18a
Rickets in a 3-month-old infant.

Figure 18b
Healing after 28 days of vitamin D treatment.

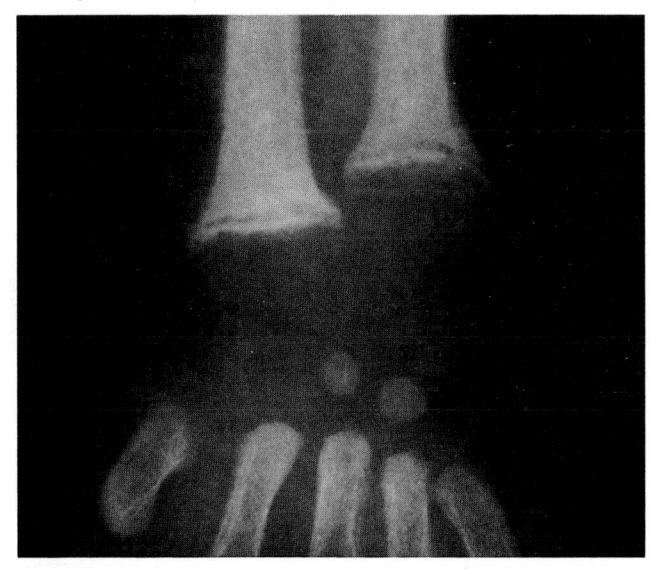

Figure 18c
After 41 days. In these photographs no shadow is cast by the epiphyses, which are still unossified.

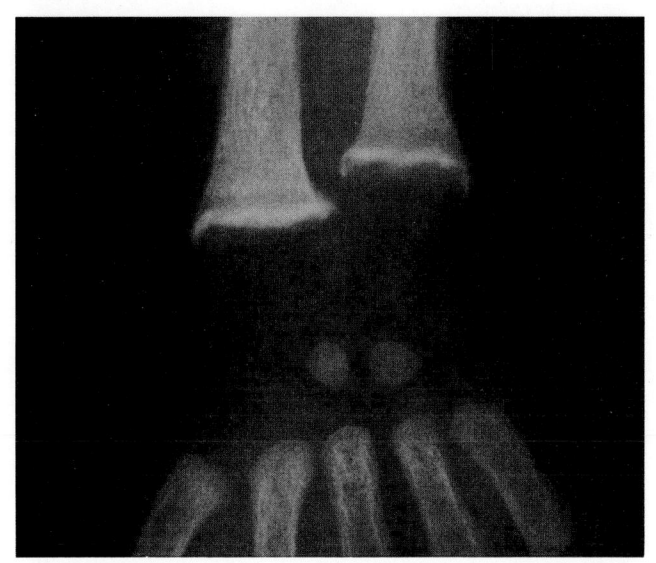

Rickets is recognized by X-ray most readily in the wrist. The uncalcified lower ends of the bones are porous, ragged, and saucer-shaped.

on the affected bones. Deformities occur later, especially in the pelvis and spine. The patient may walk with his feet widely spaced and may appear to waddle. Spontaneous fractures often are a complication of severe osteomalacia. In some cases tetany develops and may be seen as involuntary twitchings of the muscles of the face and by carpopedal spasms.

Diagnosis

Radiographs will show extensive demineralization, bony deformities and if present, fractures. The level of serum alkaline phosphatase is raised above the maximum normal adult level of 5 Bodansky units and the concentration of serum calcium often decreases below 8 mg./100 ml.

Treatment

Vitamin D, 125 μg. (50,000 I.U.) daily should be given as a vitamin preparation. Calcium is easily provided as milk if available; otherwise some other form such as calcium lactate is adequate. Freedom of the exposed skin to sunlight should be encouraged. Good obstetrical care is very important in women who have pelvic abnormalities due to osteomalacia.

Endemic Goiter

Goiter is the name used for any swelling of the thyroid gland. When it occurs sporadically it may be due to a number of different causes not related to diet and not, therefore, relevant to this monograph. However, where goiter is common or endemic in a district or in a community, the cause is usually nutritional, due to a lack of the mineral nutrient iodine.

In endemic goiter areas, frequently many people have some enlargement of the thyroid gland and a smaller number have large and obvious swellings of the neck. By far the commonest cause of endemic goiter is a deficiency of iodine in the diet of those affected. The amount of iodine present in soil varies from place to place and this affects the quantity both in food grown and in the water supply of the area.

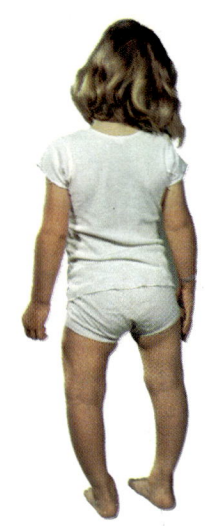

Figure 17b
Back view of same child.

the bone becomes coarse and there is a decrease in bone density. Curvature of the bones may be even more evident in radiographs than is found in clinical examination, especially in a plump child. Some of the early radiographic changes in rickets are rather similar to those of infantile scurvy.

The serum alkaline phosphatase is usually elevated well above the normal range of 5-15 Bodansky units. A level above 20 units in a child is very suggestive of rickets. The serum phosphorus is usually reduced to 2-4 mg./100 ml. (normal = 4.5-5.5 mg./100 ml.), but the serum calcium is frequently normal or only slightly reduced, being around 10 mg./100 ml.

Treatment

The basis of treatment is the provision of adequate quantities of vitamin D at the same time ensuring an adequate intake of calcium. Vitamin preparations that provide about 75 µg. (3000 I.U.) of vitamin D daily is the recommended therapy. Calcium supplementation is usually given as milk.

Simultaneously with treatment the mother should be educated regarding the value of sunshine on the body as well as given good nutritional instruction.

Mild bony deformities tend to right themselves following dietary treatment, but in more serious cases some degree of deformity may persist.

Osteomalacia

Osteomalacia is the adult counterpart of rickets and has the same general causes. It occurs much more frequently in women than in men. It is most common in women on a poor diet who have been depleted of calcium by many years of pregnancies and lactation, who get very little vitamin D in their diet and who are protected from the sun by their clothing and confinement indoors. The condition is usually very rare in the U.S.

The Disease

Pain occurs in the bones of the pelvis, lower back and the legs. Tenderness may be elicited by pressure

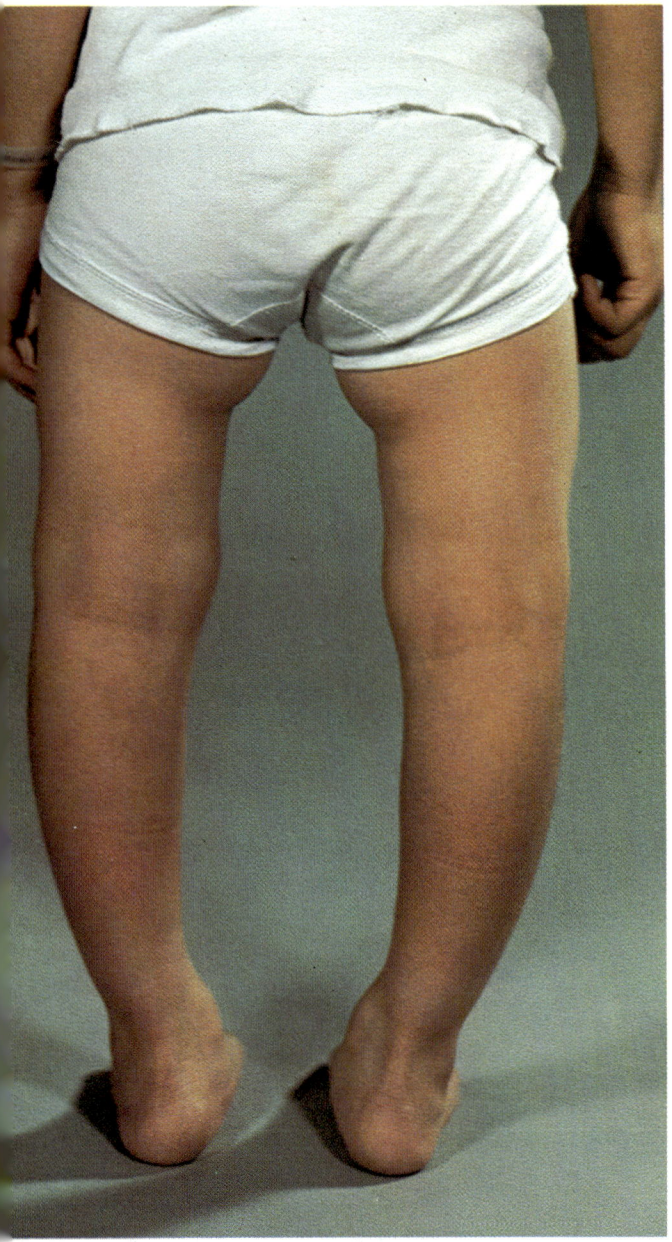

Figure 17c
Close-up from back, note angle of feet.

creased gradually to 2 gr. daily. Weight loss, increased pulse rate and a raised BMR are indications of hyperthyroidism and are a signal to reduce the dosage.

Surgical treatment consisting of sub-total thyroidectomy is indicated for large goiters, especially the adenomatous type and for those exceptional cases that do not respond to iodine or thyroid extract.

Prevention of endemic goiter

Where goiter is prevalent it constitutes a public health problem and should be tackled as such. The most satisfactory measure is the addition of iodide to all salt sold in the area. This will reduce the size of many existing goiters ad will prevent most goiters from developing in the future.

Salt is most commonly iodized with sodium or potassium iodide to a level which provides about 0.5 grams of iodine to 1 kilogram of salt. The less volatile potassium iodate is preferable to iodide for iodination in hot, humid countries or regions. When endemic goiter is a problem it is desirable to pass legislation to ensure that all salt is iodized. Unfortunately legislation does not now exist throughout the U.S. or in most states to require the iodinization of all table salt or salt used in processed foods. Iodized and noniodized salt is available in stores, displayed side by side, and there is recent evidence of increasing iodine deficiency in the U.S. This is really inexcusable.

Figure 20
Goiter in a young woman.

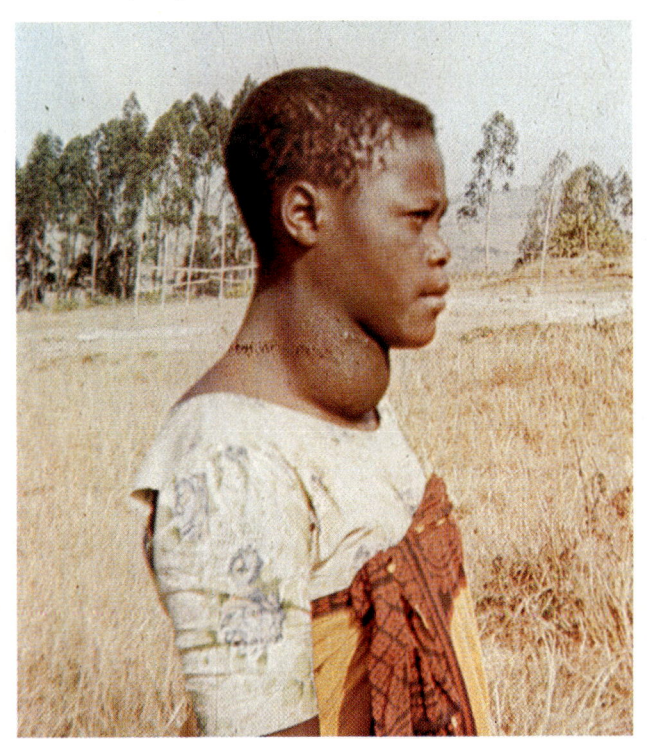

Figure 21
Advanced nodular goiters in an endemic area in Tanzania.

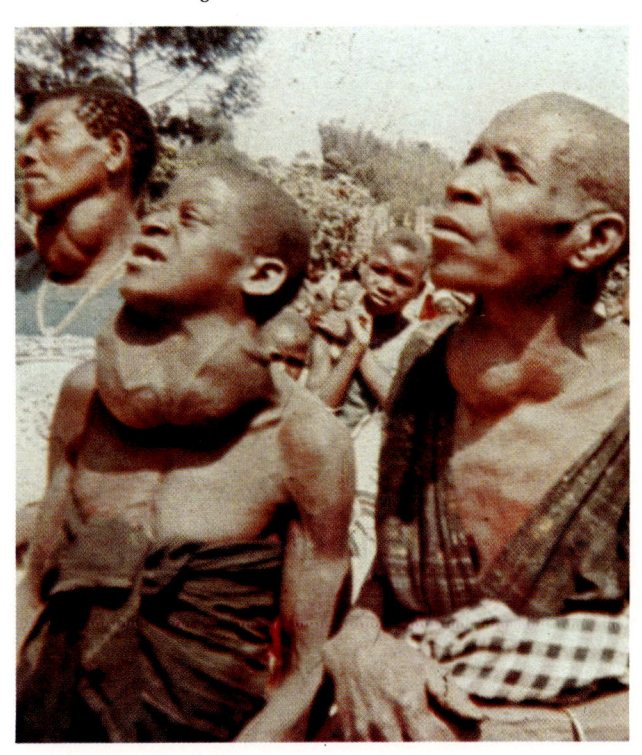

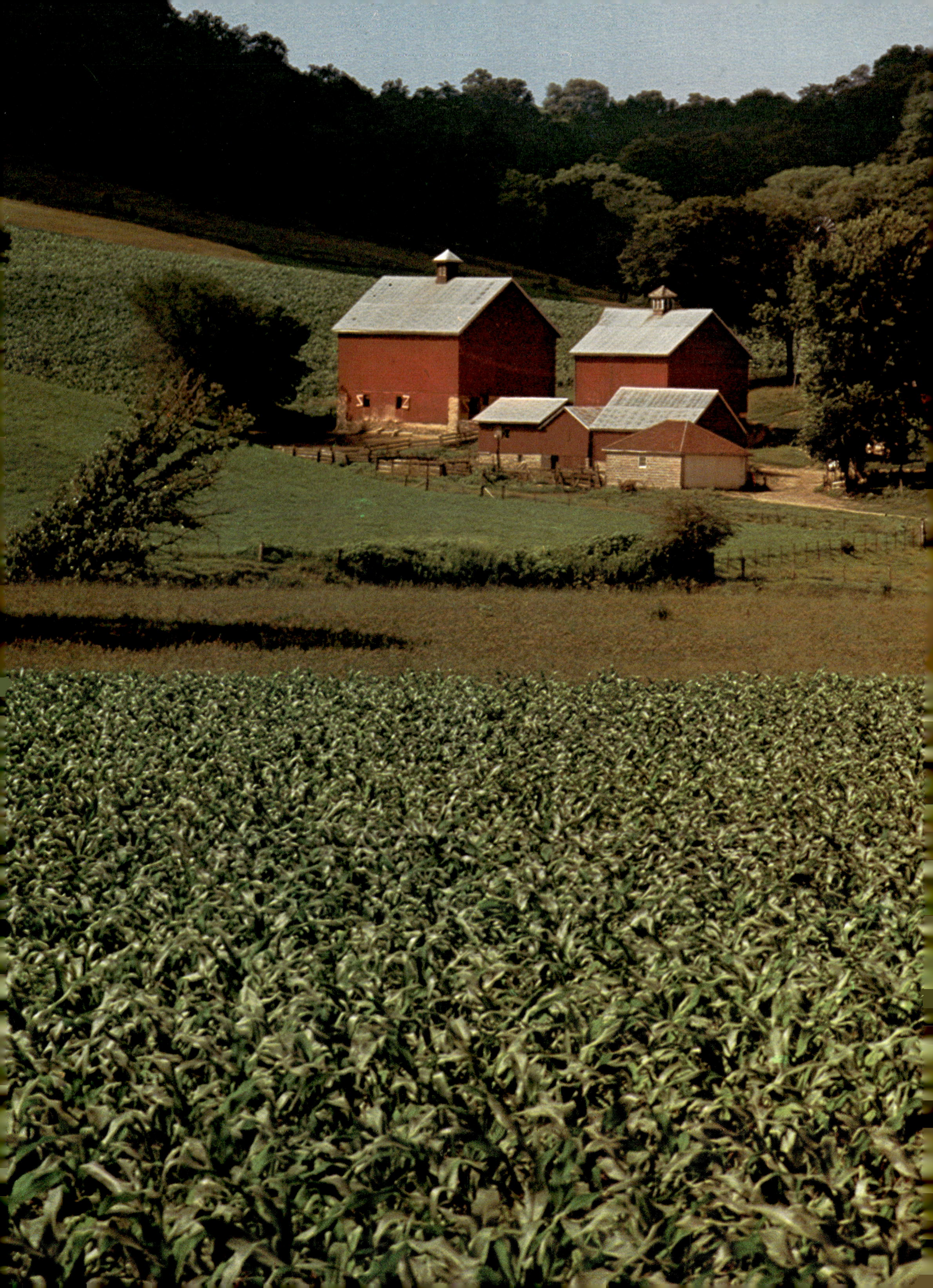

Nutrients

Protein

Dietary proteins furnish the necessary sources of amino acids and nitrogen for synthesis of body proteins and the array of other nitrogen-containing compounds excepting the nitrogen-containing vitamins. Most of the dietary protein is utilized as amino acids and absorbed by the intestinal mucosa after hydrolysis of complex peptide chains. Some twenty-two amino acids are of biological importance. Of these, eight so-called essential amino acids cannot be synthesized by man in amounts necessary for his needs.[29] These are lysine, leucine, isoleucine, methionine, phenylalanine, threonine, tryptophan, and valine. In addition, an exogenous supply of histidine is necessary for early growth and development. Requirements for the other amino acids are met either through exogenous sources or endogenous sources through synthesis from appropriate metabolic precursors and exogenous amino nitrogen.

Dietary proteins are supplied by both animal and plant materials. The nutritional quality of proteins from various sources is a function of the particular amino acids they contain in relation to essential amino acid requirements.

In general, protein from animal sources is of greater nutritional value because it contains all of the essential amino acids plus the non-essential ones. Proteins from cereals and vegetables are relatively deficient in certain amino acids, particularly lysine, tryptophan, threonine and methionine, depending on the specific cereal or vegetable and in addition provide less of all the essential amino acids per unit weight of protein than do those from animal sources. On the other hand, relatively small amounts of a high quality animal protein can efficiently supplement the relative amino acid deficiencies in diets obtained mainly from plant protein. Similarly appropriate mixtures of cereals, legumes or other vegetable foods may have a protein quality approaching that of animal foods.

In adults there is little if any absorption of peptide chains. The amino acids themselves are absorbed by an active transport system against a concentration gradient. Specificities in the transfer sites lead to differential rates of absorption and to competition in the transport of amino acids across the intestinal mucosa. A similar transfer system operates in other cells as well. There is no known "pool"—in the usual metabolic sense—of amino acids. And so a continuing, normal level of protein synthesis requires the continuous availability of the entire array of necessary amino acids. The removal of even one essential amino acid from the diet leads rather rapidly to a lower level of protein synthesis in the body.

Minimal protein requirements for a healthy adult represent the sum of the requirements for the essential amino acids plus sufficient utilizable nitrogen to maintain overall synthesis of nitrogen containing molecules. Nitrogen loss occurs in the urine, the feces, the skin, hair, and nails. Though there are considerable problems in measuring minimal protein requirement, it is of the order of 0.3 to 0.4 gm. protein/kg./day, assuming a reasonable amount of high quality protein or an appropriate mixture of cereal or vegetable protein with an adequate level of overall calories. With lower quality proteins, greater quantities are required to maintain nitrogen balance. Early growth and development, pregnancy, lactation, and periods of physical stress add to the basal requirement for protein. Recommended allowances include a two-to-three-fold "safety factor" over minimal requirements and apply to the ranges of quality in mixed proteins ordinarily consumed.

It is the very high (on a body weight basis) requirement for protein during early growth and development which makes this age group especially vulnerable to dietary deprivation.

In addition, the sometimes very marked degradation of protein and excretion of urinary nitrogen which accompanies the stress of even ordinarily mild childhood illnesses, puts such an added burden on an

---

29. Rose, W. C., *Federation Proc.* 8:546, 1949.

already tenuously nourished infant that it can start the spiral to frank, clinical malnutrition.

Carbohydrate

Carbohydrates comprise the major energy source for populations throughout the world and, being derived from foods readily and efficiently grown in nearly all climates, are cheaper than animal proteins and fats. The carbohydrate contribution to total daily calories is about 45% in the diets of people in highly developed areas. Whereas for the ⅞ of the world's population that rely mainly on plants as sources of food, this contribution amounts to about 70% and may be as high as 90%.

The common hexoses—glucose, fructose, galactose, and mannose—are the digestion products absorbed from the gastrointestinal hydrolysis of the di- and polysaccharides occuring in foods.

In affluent societies about half the dietary carbohydrate is furnished by starches and dextrins (both polysaccharides of glucose units), 25 to 30% by sucrose (glucose and fructose), the rest from lactose, glucose, fructose, and an array of only partly digestible polysaccharides. In less developed areas the proportionate contributions of the various types of carbohydrate are quite different. Sucrose and lactose (glucose and galactose) are consumed in much smaller quantities, while starches and other complex polysaccharides make up most of the total dietary carbohydrate. A trend in American diets over the past fifty years is marked by the decreasing consumption of starches from cereals and vegetables and an increased *per capita* utilization of refined sucrose. On the other hand, unrefined complex carbohydrate foods from cereals and vegetables substantially contribute to the vitamin and mineral intake in many areas of the world where they provide the major source of calories. Although these sources may be relatively less important in ordinary American diets, the increased reliance on refined carbohydrates does produce constraints on the achievement of adequate nutrient intakes in very low-calorie diets.

There are no specific requirements established for carbohydrates as to type, source or amount. During starvation and with calorie restricted diets, carbohydrate can serve to spare body proteins for energy purposes; as little as 100 gm. per day (400 calories) of carbohydrates can prevent the water and electrolyte loss attendant with protein catabolism, and probably as little as 40 gm. per day are necessary to prevent the development of ketosis.

Fats

Fats and oils in nutrition have historically been associated with the energy or caloric value of a diet and with its satiety value. This is because they provide twice as many calories per unit of weight as either carbohydrate or protein (9 calories per gram versus 4) and because most people enjoy the taste of fats as they are characteristically used in our diets. Because fats remain in the stomach appreciably longer than carbohydrates or proteins, they tend to give a feel of "gastronomic satisfaction" for a somewhat longer period of time. More recently the interest in fats has been less on their caloric and satiety properties and more on their influence on the level of cholesterol in the blood and their association with atherosclerosis.

About 98% of dietary fats are triglycerides or compounds of glycerol and specific fatty acids. Since glycerol has three hydroxyl groups, each of which can combine with a fatty acid, we speak of triglycerides, diglycerides, and monoglycerides depending upon how many of the hydroxyl groups of the glycerol molecule have been esterified with a fatty acid. Additionally these fatty acids may be saturated, monounsaturated, or polyunsaturated. The term "saturation" refers to the degree of hydrogenation of the carbon atoms of the fatty acid chain. When all of the carbon atoms of the fatty acid chain are attached to the maximum number of hydrogen atoms, the chain is "saturated" with hydrogen–a saturated fat. If the carbon chain has one double bond and hence can accept two more hydrogen atoms, we call the fat monounsaturated. If the carbon chain has two or more double bonds and thus can accept four or more hydrogen atoms, we call the fat polyunsaturated. As previously stated all naturally occurring fats are mixtures of saturated, monounsaturated, and polyunsaturated fats, but the mixtures vary widely in composition. Thus, butter averages 66% saturates, 31% monounsaturates, and 3% polyunsaturates. Soybean oil averages 15% saturates, 25% monounsaturates, and 60% polyunsaturates while safflower oil has a still higher percentage of polyunsaturates, approximately 75% and correspondingly lower amount of monounsaturates and saturates.

In the processes of digestion, fats are mostly hydrolyzed into di- and monoglycerides and fatty acids by the action of various enzymes–lipases. As these lipases are present in pancreatic and intestinal juices, most of the digestion of fat takes place in the upper part of the small intestine. In the small intestine the fats are emulsified by the bile and this process facilitates the enzymatic action of the various lipases. Ordinarily most 12-carbon and longer fatty acids upon being emulsified and hydrolyzed, are absorbed into the lymphatic system and transported in association with cholesterol, phospholipids, and protein; these particles are termed chylomicrons. The chylomicrons then undergo a process of dissolution brought about by the action of an enzyme lipoprotein, lipase, found in blood and tissue.

In recent years finely divided and stable emulsions of fat have been prepared which may be given intravenously. Such emulsions are metabolized similarly to fat which has been eaten and they serve a useful role when complete intravenous nutrition is necessary for periods of several weeks.

Because the level of cholesterol in the blood is one of the factors associated with the development of coronary heart disease and other manifestations of atherosclerosis, and as the type of dietary fat is an important factor influencing the level of cholesterol in the blood, interest in fat has greatly increased in recent years. In general, the saturated fats increase the level of blood cholesterol, the monounsaturated fats have no effect, and the polyunsaturated fats decrease the cholesterol level. There is as yet no clear biochemical explanation for these regulating effects.

The common saturated fats of our diet are milk fat, meat fat, butter, cream, most cheese and coconut oil. Olive and peanut oils are examples of oils in which the predominant fats are monounsaturated. Safflower, soya, corn and cottonseed oils are the common oils in which the predominant fat is polyunsaturated because of the linoleic acid they contain. A diet designed to lower the level of cholesterol in the blood is low in saturated fat and high in polyunsaturated fat (see Section on Cardiovascular Disease).

The four commonly used polyunsaturated vegetable oils average 50% or more linoleic acid (safflower oil is 70% linoleic acid). In the preparation of these oils for commercial use in products such as shortenings and margarine and to give the oils greater stability, they are partially hydrogenated. This, of course, reduces their polyunsaturation and increases their saturation. But, hydrogenation is a controllable process. One can hydrogenate a lot or a little. Thus, a vegetable oil, 50% of which consisted of the polyunsaturated fatty acid, linoleic, may have been hydrogenated in the process of making margarine so that the polyunsaturation has been reduced to 35 to 40%, but the final product is still a good source of linoleic acid when compared with lard at about 9% polyunsaturated and with butter at less than 3% of polyunsaturates.

An additional component of dietary fat which influences the level of blood lipids is dietary cholesterol. The level of consumption of egg yolk, butterfat, and meat fats in the usual American diet provides from 600 to 800 mg. daily of exogenous cholesterol

Figure 22
Photomicrograph of crystals of human ferritin.

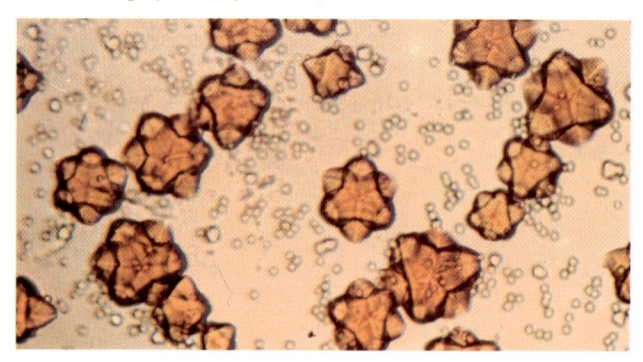

with egg yolks alone contributing more than one-half of the total. Foods rich in cholesterol are also restricted in planning fat-modified diets.

Water

Because water forms somewhat more than 60% of the body weight of man, it obviously plays an important part in metabolism. Except for fat storage the whole series of chemical actions that are intimately related to the life of a living organism, animal or vegetable, are ultimately referable to changes that take place in solution. It has been shown that the younger the animal, the richer it is in water. It has also been found that the fatter the animal, the smaller the percentage of water.

Water serves as a solvent to help absorb water-soluble nutrients and eliminate water-soluble waste products via the urine. It is indispensable for the control of body temperature via the evaporation of water from the lungs and from the skin.

Water furnishes no calories or vitamins, but it may provide various minerals—calcium and magnesium in the case of hard water and fluoride in the case of waters that have been fluoridated either naturally or by man.

Under normal conditions, 6 or 7 eight-ounce glasses of fluid (water, tea, coffee, etc.) furnish enough water for the metabolic needs of the tissues of adults. The human being can live far longer without food than he can without water.

Minerals

IRON

The average iron content of a healthy adult is only about 4 grams and yet this relatively small quantity is vitally important.[30] Iron deficiency anemia is a common cause of ill health in the United States and in all parts of the world.

About two-thirds of the iron in the body is present in the blood mainly as hemoglobin and approximately 3% is present as myoglobin. The majority of the remainder is storage iron which is found in the liver, spleen, bone marrow and muscle in the form of ferritin or hemosiderin. Additional minute quantities exist in the respiratory enzymes and in iron-binding protein of the plasma.

The main function of iron is its vital role in the transfer of oxygen at various sites in the body. Iron is an essential component of hemoglobin, the pigment in the red blood cells which carries oxygen from the lungs to the tissues. Iron is present as myoglobin in skeletal and heart muscle where it functions by accepting the oxygen from the hemoglobin and also in peroxidase, catalase and the cytochromes.

Iron is not an element which tends to be either used up or destroyed in the properly functioning body. Unlike some minerals it is not required for excretion and only very small amounts appear in the urine and sweat. Minute quantities are lost in desquamated cells from the skin and intestine, in shed hair and nails and in the bile and other body secretions. The body is however, efficiently economical and conservative in the use of iron. Iron which is released when the erythrocytes are old and broken down is taken up and utilized again and again for the manufacture of new red blood cells. This economy with iron is important. In normal circumstances only about 1 milligram of iron is lost to the body daily by excretion into the intestines, in urine, in sweat or through loss of hair or surface epithelial cells.

Because of the preservation of iron, the nutritional needs of healthy males and post-menopausal females are very small. Women of childbearing age must however, make good the iron lost during menstruation and childbirth and meet the additional requirements

30. Drabkin, D. L., *Physiol. Revs. 31*:345, 1951.

of pregnancy and lactation. Children have relatively high needs because of their rapid growth which not only increases their body size but also their blood volume.

Sources of iron

Iron is present in a great variety of foods, of both plant and animal origin. In many individual foods there is a considerable variation in the value of iron content according to the soil and other conditions in which the food is raised. Rich food sources for iron include meat, especially liver, egg yolk and pulses such as beans and peas. However, many other common foods such as green leafy vegetables, whole grain and enriched cereals, vegetables and fish are good sources of iron. Milk, both human and cow's, contrary to the notion that it is the "perfect food," is a poor source of iron.

In the United States many prepared foods such as bread, breakfast cereals and certain baby foods are artificially enriched with iron. An average American adult diet consisting of a variety of common foods bought at a supermarket or grocery store or eaten in a restaurant or institution would normally contain about 15 milligrams of iron per day. Because of the poor absorption of iron this may be a rather marginal amount.

Absorption of iron

The absorption of iron takes place mainly in the upper portion of the small intestine. Most of the iron enters the blood stream directly and not via the lymphatics. The precise mechanism by which this absorption takes place across the mucosal cells is not known. Evidence indicates that absorption is regulated to some extent by physiological demand. The important factors may be iron stores, hypoxia, erythropoietic activity and level of unsaturated iron-binding protein. Thus, persons who are iron-deficient tend to absorb iron more efficiently and in greater quantities than do normal subjects. This phenomenon has been demonstrated both with medicinal ferrous sulphate and with food tagged with radioactive Fe^{59}.

There are several other factors which affect iron absorption. For example, phosphates and phytates in food reduce while ascorbic acid increases iron absorption. Malabsorption syndromes and gastrectomy reduce, whereas pyridoxine deficiency, untreated pernicious anemia and chronic pancreatic insufficiency increase the absorption of iron. A recent report suggests that egg yolk, despite its relatively large amount of iron, inhibits the absorption of iron.[31]

The availability of the iron in foodstuffs is very variable. Healthy subjects normally absorb only 5 to 10 per cent of the iron in their foods whereas iron-deficient subjects may absorb twice this amount. Therefore on a diet consisting of 15 milligrams of iron, 0.75 to 1.5 milligrams of iron would be absorbed in a normal subject but as much as 3 milligrams in an iron-deficient subject. Similarly absorption is generally increased during growth and pregnancy, following bleeding and in other conditions where an enhanced demand for iron exists.

Requirements

From the foregoing it will be clear that dietary requirements of iron are in the order of ten times the body's physiologic requirements. Thus, if a normal man or post-menopausal woman requires 1 milligram of iron daily due to iron losses then the dietary requirements are about 10 milligrams per day. This may allow a fair margin of safety especially as absorption is increased with need.

Menstrual loss of iron has been estimated to average a little under 1 milligram per day taken over the whole year.[32] The recommendation is that females of child bearing age have a dietary intake of 18 milligrams per day.

The average daily iron requirements necessary to develop the fetus and tissues and to expand the maternal blood supply during pregnancy is about 1.5

---

31. Symposium: Iron Deficiency and Absorption, *Am. J. Clin. Nutr.* 21:1138, 1968.
32. Frenchman, R. and Johnston, F. A., *J. Am. Dietet. Assoc.* 25:217, 1949.

milligrams. Most of this additional iron is required in the second and third trimesters of pregnancy.

Satisfactory studies have not been made regarding iron requirements or rate of iron absorption during lactation. Human breast milk contains only about 0.2 milligrams iron per 100 milliliters, so that a woman in full lactation might be losing 1 milligram or more of iron per day in her milk.

Infants are born with a store of iron which is adequate for the first three months of life. Premature infants may have a reduced iron store at birth and are therefore more liable to develop iron-deficiency anemia. Recommended daily dietary allowances of iron range from 6 milligrams at age 1 month, up to 15 milligrams for those 1 to 3 years old.

Iron deficiency

A glance at the nutritional requirements for iron and the iron content of commonly eaten foods might suggest that iron deficiency should be very rare in persons on a normal diet except during pregnancy and lactation. This is probably true of the "normal" subject. However, iron loss occurs whenever blood loss occurs. A very frequent cause of iron deficiency anemia is a chronic loss of blood about which the patient may be unaware or unconcerned. This may result for example from mild peptic ulcer, from bleeding gums or hemorrhoids, from menorrhagia, from hookworm infestation and in the tropics from schistosomiasis especially of the urinary tract. Whenever blood is lost, iron is lost and if not replaced it will lead to iron-deficiency anemia. This condition is described with other anemias on page 27.

Iron excess

Hemosiderosis is a condition in which excessive accumulations of iron have occurred in the human due to a number of causes. These have included frequent blood transfusions, especially for hemolytic anemia (in this condition the erythrocytes are destroyed but their iron is not lost to the body) and from excessive oral or parenteral doses of therapeutic iron or as a result of excessive consumption of iron in food. For example the diet of Bantu natives of South Africa contains quantities of iron often exceeding 100 mg. per day—the result of using iron utensils in their daily cooking and for the preparation of fermented beverages.[33] It is also seen in hemochromatosis, a disease believed to be due to an inborn error of metabolism in which excessive iron is absorbed from the diet. The danger of excessive ingestion of medicinal iron is constantly present, especially as enthusiastic advertising leads the health-conscious layman to believe that iron is a body strengthener and a tonic. This may result in persons believing that the more that is taken the better for his or her health. A large variety of iron containing medicinal preparations are available without prescription and there are many foods fortified with iron. As a result it is common for persons to be consuming many times the recommended allowances for iron. Accidental poisoning with ferrous sulphate has sometimes been fatal in children.

In iron overload, the plasma iron content is high, the iron binding capacity is depressed and the per cent saturation is nearly complete.

CALCIUM AND PHOSPHORUS

Although calcium and phosphorus are not chemically related they occur together in the body in a ratio that is nearly constant. About 1.5 per cent of the human body is composed of calcium and 1 per cent of phosphorus. These two minerals are mainly in the bones where the calcium combines with phosphorus as various calcium phosphate salts to form a hard substance which gives the body rigidity. However, the skeleton of the body is not the rigid unchanging structure which it appears to be. In fact the bones contain a cellular matrix and calcium is continuously taken up by the bones and given back to the body. The bones also function as a reservoir for these minerals. Appreciable loss or gain in calcium is usually reflected in similar changes in phosphorus content.

33. Bothwell, T. H. and Bradlow, B. A., *Arch. Path.* 70:279, 1960.

Calcium

The body of a healthy adult contains about 1250 grams of calcium, 99 per cent of which is in the bones and teeth. Calcium is present in the blood serum in small but important quantities, usually about 10 mg. in 100 ml. of serum. A substantial reduction in this amount causes the development of tetany while an increase may lead to respiratory or cardiac failure due to impaired muscle function. Approximately 60 per cent of serum calcium is ionized while the remainder is bound to serum proteins. The extra-cellular fluids and soft tissues of an adult contain approximately 10 grams of calcium.

Sources

A great variety of foods such as whole grain cereal products, leafy vegetables, legumes and nuts contain calcium with particularly rich sources being milk and cheese. Sardines and other small fish in which the bones are eaten are other important sources of calcium.

Cow's milk contains 120 mg./100 ml., considerably more than human breast milk (30 mg./100 ml.).

Absorption

Calcium absorption depends on several factors but vitamin D is one of the most important. Thus, even if the intake of calcium is adequate, calcium absorption is reduced and calcium balance may be negative if the subject is deficient in vitamin D.

Certain amino acids, citric acid and lactose enhance calcium absorption. In contrast, phosphates, phytates and oxalates inhibit calcium absorption. It is doubtful, however, if any of these substances are ordinarily important determinants of the calcium requirements of man.

Of considerable importance in calcium metabolism and calcium requirements is the human power of adaptation. The physical basis of adaptation is not proven but its existence is clear.

People eating low calcium diets have been shown to have a more efficient absorption of calcium than those customarily eating diets higher in calcium. Thus as the intake of calcium is lowered the efficiency of the body to absorb and retain calcium increases, while raising calcium intake results in reduced utilization.

Calcium is present in the feces, urine and sweat, that in the feces being primarily dietary calcium which for a number of reasons has not been absorbed. The amount of calcium in the urine varies greatly but usually is that which has been absorbed but not taken up by the skeleton or soft tissues. Considerable quantities of calcium may be lost in sweat in individuals working at high temperatures.

Requirements

A specific statement of man's calcium requirement is not easy to make because of the "adaptation mechanism," the many other factors influencing absorption, and the variability in calcium loss from the body. The recommended allowances (NAS/NRC 1968) are put at 800 mg. calcium daily for adults, a figure well above theoretical estimates of need.

The FAO/WHO Expert Group[34] suggested that a practical allowance for adults would be an intake of 400 to 500 mg. daily.

Additional calcium is needed during pregnancy and lactation. The fetus has its calcium needs and human breast milk contains merely 30 mg. calcium per 100 ml. Therefore, during pregnancy and lactation an extra allowance of 500 mg. calcium is recommended above the normal adult requirements. Without this the woman is likely to deplete her own calcium reserves.

Children are constantly increasing the size of their skeletons and so have especially high calcium requirements. The recommended dietary allowances are put at 700 mg. for infants (which incidentally is higher than the amount which would be obtained from breast milk) and rises to 1400 mg. daily during the pubertal growth spurt and the teen age period.

34. *Calcium Requirements*, World Health Organization Technical Reports Series No. 230, WHO, Geneva, 1961.

Deficiency

Despite the publicity given to the importance of a high calcium intake and the scientific work done on calcium requirements in adult man there is no convincing evidence to show that a deficiency of calcium even at levels of 250 to 300 mg. daily is harmful. Presumably adults achieve balance at the level of intake supplied by their usual diet, largely because of "adaptation."

In females on a habitually low calcium intake, depletion of body calcium resulting from repeated pregnancies and prolonged lactation may play a role in the development of osteomalacia. However, vitamin D deficiency is far more often implicated in this condition.

Even in children the development of rickets is known to be largely independent of calcium intake. There is still no convincing evidence on whether low calcium intakes, so commonly found in developing countries, adversely affect the growth of children.

Osteoporosis is a common disease of aging in the United States and in many other parts of the world. Loss of bone may be an inevitable process of aging and usually starts in middle age. Although high calcium diets are frequently recommended in osteoporosis and in the diets of the elderly there is not good scientific evidence to show that this measure actually increases bone density. There is now evidence to show that a high intake of fluoride benefits calcium retention in osteoporosis.

Excess

Certain populations such as the Masai in East Africa who consume a diet almost exclusively of milk may have intakes of over 2000 mg. calcium per day. This has not been shown to have any deleterious effects.

However, there are conditions in which excessive calcium is found in the serum, urine or soft tissues such as idiopathic hypercalcemia, the "milk alkali syndrome," renal stone formation, hypercalciuria and fluorosis. At the present time there are no epidemiologic data to prove that high calcium intakes are responsible for these conditions.

IODINE

The body of an average adult contains about 40 mg. of iodine of which about half is present in the thyroid gland. Iodine is essential for the formation of thyroxine and triiodothyronine, the hormones of this gland.

Sources

Iodine is present in rocks and soils but through the ages much has been washed into the sea. Man gets his iodine from food and from water, which vary in amount according to the iodine content of their source. Thus there are waters with a fairly high content of iodine and others with negligible amounts, and the same foodstuff grown in different soils has a different iodine content.

Seafoods on the whole are rich in iodine and dairy products, eggs, and some vegetables may be good sources. Iodized salt is sold in the United States but housewives are frequently unaware as to whether they are buying iodized or non-iodized salt and even institutions such as hospitals and schools are frequently found to be using non-iodized salt, a most unfortunate situation.

The Food and Nutrition Board of our National Research Council has recommended federal legislation making mandatory the iodization of all salt put up for sale for human consumption. However, there is as yet no federal legislation concerning salt, and state laws are not uniform. A suitable iodine level is 0.5 gram of potassium iodide in 1 kilogram of purified salt.

Absorption and utilization

In normal people, iodine is readily absorbed from the intestinal tract and about one third is utilized by the thyroid gland while two thirds is excreted in the urine. Iodine nutriture can be studied by determining the avidity of the thyroid gland to take up radioactive iodine, by measurement of the stable iodine content of the urine, and by determination of the protein-bound iodine. Iodine in the feces comes mainly from the bile.

Requirements

It has been suggested that 1 microgram of iodine per kilogram body weight is an adequate intake in the human. However, growing children and women during pregnancy and lactation have increased needs.

Deficiency

A deficiency of iodine leads to the development of goiter but there are several other causes of goiter besides iodine deficiency. Endemic goiter which is discussed on page 48 occurs where population groups have dietary sources of iodine below normal requirements. Iodine lack is a major public health problem in many parts of the world[35] as well as in the U.S. due to our laxness in using iodized salt.

Iodine deficiency goiter is really a defense mechanism designed to keep thyroid hormones at an optimal level. A decrease in the circulating iodine-containing thyroid hormones triggers a release of thyroid-stimulating hormone (TSH) from the pituitary gland. This eventually causes a thyroid hypertrophy and an increase in the number of thyroid epithelial cells.

Goitrogens in brassica plants such as cabbage have been shown to increase the needs of iodine in certain laboratory animals. As a result iodine intakes which would be adequate under normal circumstances failed to prevent goiter in those animals consuming large quantities of goitrogens. There is little evidence to show that goitrogens in normal diets have been important in the production of goiter in man.

FLUORIDE

In man fluoride deposition is found mainly in the teeth and the skeleton but the total quantity is small. However the presence of traces of this mineral in the teeth helps to protect them against caries and as such,

35. Follis, R. H., J. Trop. Med. Hyg. 12:137, 1964.

Chart 7
Missing Teeth per Adult
(fluoride and non-fluoride communities)

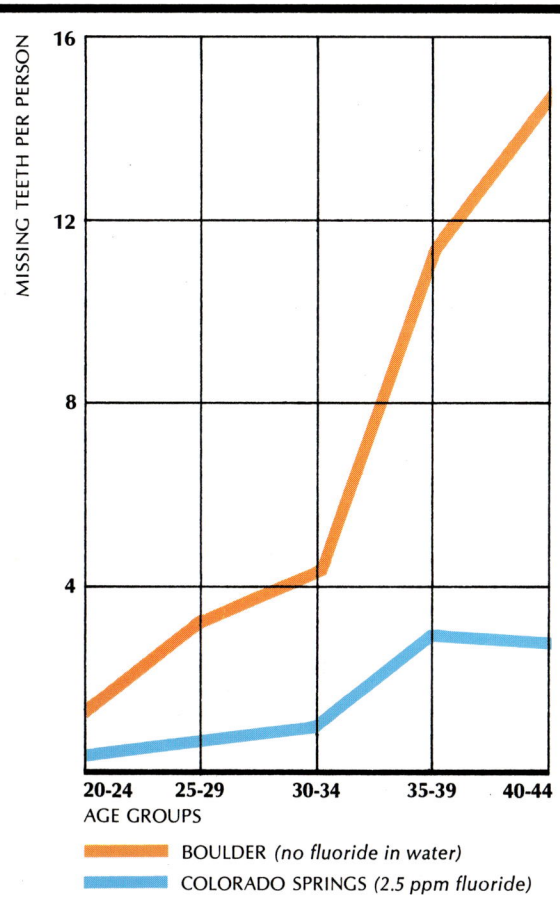

BOULDER *(no fluoride in water)*
COLORADO SPRINGS *(2.5 ppm fluoride)*

That the benefits of fluoride accrued during childhood are carried over into adulthood is shown by a comparision of missing teeth of adults in Boulder, Colorado (no fluoride in the drinking water) and Colorado Springs (2.5 ppm of fluoride in the drinking water). At age 40-44 the loss of teeth is less than 4 permanent teeth per person in Colorado Springs while it averages about 16 permanent teeth loss per person in Boulder, Colorado. The ratio of tooth loss is 4 to 5 times greater, at all times, in the non-fluoride area than in the fluoride area from age 20 to 44.

Chart 8
Dental Caries and Dental Fluorosis in relation to fluoride in public water supplies.

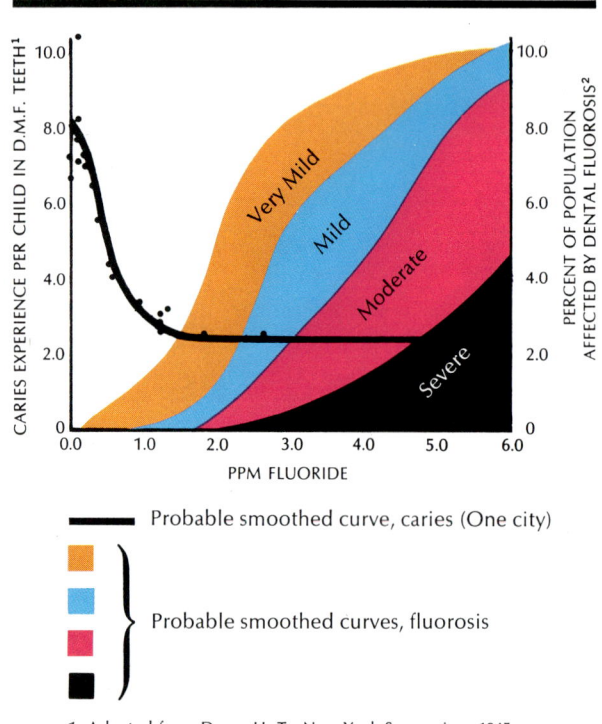

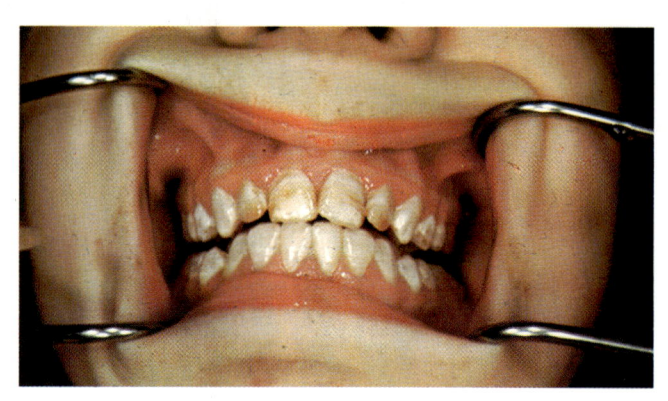

— Probable smoothed curve, caries (One city)

} Probable smoothed curves, fluorosis

1. Adapted from Dean, H. T., New York Symposium 1945.
2. Adapted from Dean, H. T., Int. Den. J. 4:311-337, 1954.

Figure 23
Mild fluorosis shown as mottling of the permanent teeth. This 14-year-old drank well water containing 5.5 ppm of fluoride from birth.

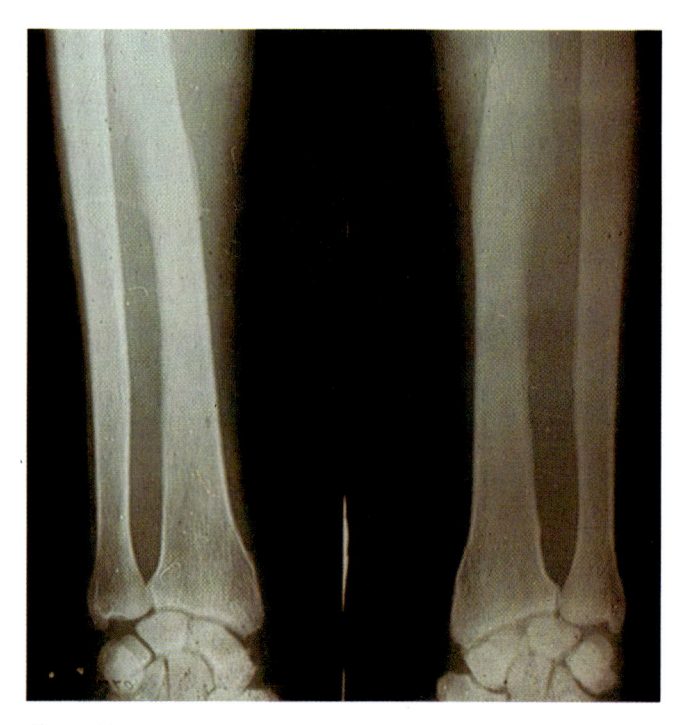

Figure 24
Skeletal fluorosis. This resulted from prolonged consumption of water from a stream containing 18 ppm of fluoride. X-ray of forearm shows calcific deposits between the radius and ulna.

Human Requirements

The Food and Nutrition Board's (7th Ed. 1968) Recommended Daily Allowance for adults is 1.5 mg. (5000 I.U.) and is considered to be provided by 1.2 mg. (4000 I.U.) of beta-carotene and 0.3 mg. (1000 units) of pre-formed vitamin A. Allowances of vitamin A for infants and children are somewhat more liberal in terms of recommended allowances in order to provide for growth and to ensure adequate body stores. For the second and third trimester of pregnancy an added daily allowance of 0.3 mg. (1000 I.U.) and for lactation an added daily allowance of 0.9 mg. (3000 I.U.) above that for the normal are recommended.

There are a number of factors which affect absorption of pro-vitamin A from the intestine. Carotene is poorly utilized in persons on a low fat diet while intestinal diseases such as dysentery, celiac disease and sprue limit the absorption of vitamin A and the conversion of carotene. Persons with obstruction of the bile ducts are likely to become deficient in vitamin A as bile salts are essential for the absorption of vitamin A and carotene.

Deficiency

A dietary deficiency of vitamin A may result in the development of xerophthalmia which may then lead to keratomalacia and blindness. This is a serious public health problem in some parts of the world. (See page 37.)

Early signs of vitamin A deficiency are night blindness and the development of dermatological lesions such as follicular hyperkeratosis and crazy pavement skin. Another sign of vitamin A deficiency, though of limited diagnostic value, are Bitot's spots which occur bilaterally in the eyes and are seen as foamy patches on the lateral side of the cornea. (See Figure 8.)

Toxicity

Hypervitaminosis of vitamin A[46] due to excessive intake has occurred with over-medication of a vitamin preparation, in faddists who include extra large doses of the vitamin in their diet, and in other circumstances where excessive amounts are taken over long periods of time.

The signs and symptoms include lethargy, malaise, abdominal pain, headaches, excessive sweating, and brittle nails. Carotenoid deposits may cause a yellow dyspigmentation of the soles of the feet, the palms of the hands and the naso-labial folds. Increased intracranial pressure and edema may develop.

THIAMINE (VITAMIN B_1)

History

The tale of Eijkman and his chickens, like the story of Jenner and his cow vaccine is a classic example of how an astute observation in an unlikely place has led to a historical landmark in the advancement of science. Working in Batavia, Java (now Djakarta, Indonesia) this Dutch physician noted that hens fed a diet of leftover rice cooked for human consumption developed a disease like beriberi. When fed either a whole grain rice or rice polishings they recovered. Eijkman[47] believed that there was a toxin present in polished rice that could be neutralized by something in rice polishings and he published his findings in 1897. In 1901 Grijns[48] first postulated that beriberi might be due to something lacking in polished rice. In 1916 McCollum and Kennedy[49] reported the finding of a water soluble B vitamin which they believed to be the anti-beriberi factor. This vitamin was subsequently divided into its anti-beriberi and anti-pellagra factors. Finally vitamin B_1, subsequently to be called thiamine, was isolated and then synthesized.

Properties

Thiamine hydrochloride is a compound consisting of a pyrimidine ring joined by a methylene bridge to a thiazole nucleus. The bond between the two rings is weak, with the result that the compound is easily destroyed in an alkaline medium. Thiamine is highly

---

46. Hillman, R. W., *Am. J. Clin. Nutr.* 4:603, 1956.
47. Eijkman, *Virchow's Archiv* 148:523, 149:187, 1897.
48. Grijns, *Tidjsch. V. Nederl. Indie* 41:3, 1901.
49. McCollum, E. V., and Kennedy, C., *J. Biol. Chem.* 24:491, 1916.

Beriberi heart.

Figure 25a
This patient was a chronic alcoholic whose diet had been poor for a long time; polyneuritis and congestive heart failure accompanied cardiac dilation. Thiamine deficiency leads to impaired function and enlargement of the heart, particularly of the right auricle and ventricle, shown by X-ray.

Figure 25b
After 1 week of thiamine therapy.

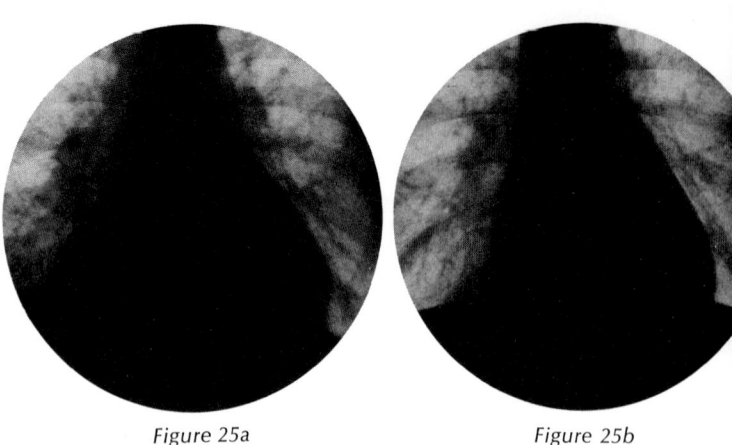

Figure 25a   *Figure 25b*

soluble in water and will resist temperatures up to 100° C. but tends to be destroyed if heated above this. This has practical implications, the vitamin being destroyed in food that is fried in a hot pan or cooked too long under pressure. Because of its solubility, thiamine is easily leached out of food-stuffs being washed or boiled.

Thiamine pyrophosphate functions in carbohydrate metabolism as a coenzyme in the decarboxylation of alpha-keto acids and in transketolase. Without cocarboxylase, pyruvic acid accumulates in various tissues, an occurrence which tends to happen in thiamine deficiency. A specific relationship between thiamine nutrition and transketolase activity at the enzyme or cellular level has likewise been observed in man.[50]

Thiamine is easily absorbed from the intestinal tract but the body is unable to store any quantity of thiamine. The liver, heart and brain have a higher concentration than muscle tissue or other organs. A person on a high thiamine intake soon becomes saturated and begins to excrete increased quantities in the urine.

Units
The activity of thiamine hydrochloride is expressed in milligrams of the chemically pure synthesized substance.

Dietary Sources
Thiamine is found in foods of both animal and vegetable origin. The richest sources among commonly eaten foods are pork, whole grain and enriched cereal grains, and the seeds of legumes. Green vegetables, fish, meat, fruit and milk all contain useful quantities.

In cereals the thiamine is present mainly in the germ and in the outer coat of the seed and much of the vitamin is lost if cereals are milled and refined.

Human Requirements
The recommended daily allowance for thiamine is 0.4 mg. per 1000 calories for all ages with an added allowance of 0.2 mg. daily during the second and third trimester of pregnancy and 0.4 mg. daily during lactation. When the daily calorie intake is less than 2000, an amount of 1.0 mg. is recommended for older adults.

Deficiency
A deficiency of thiamine is the cause of the disease beriberi. This occurs mainly among rice eating peoples and is common in Asia. In the U.S. thiamine deficiency is fairly common in alcoholics and may lead to Wernicke's disease and Korsokoff's syndrome. (See page 38.)

Toxicity
This vitamin when taken in excessive amounts is excreted in the urine and hence has no known toxicity. The kidney has no known threshold.

RIBOFLAVIN

History
Early work on the properties of vitamins in yeast and other foodstuffs showed that the antineuritic factors were destroyed by heat but that a growth promoting factor was not destroyed. This heat stable vitamin was finally isolated from milk and the yellow crystals were named riboflavin. In 1935 it was synthesized by the German chemist, Kuhn, who had also been responsible for its isolation.

Properties
Riboflavin functions as a coenzyme or active prosthetic group of flavoproteins concerned with tissue oxidation and respiration. The vitamin plays an important role in both protein and energy metabolism. Riboflavin is a water-soluble yellow crystalline substance. It is heat stable in an acid solution but decomposes in an alkaline solution or on exposure to sunlight.

50. Brin. M., *Am. J. Clin. Nutr.* 12:107, 1963.

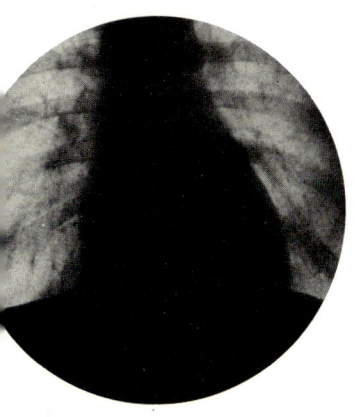

Figure 25c
After 3 weeks' treatment, progressive reduction in heart size is visible.

Figure 25c

In experimental animals a deficiency causes a failure of growth as well as lesions of the skin and eyes.

Units
Riboflavin is measured in milligrams of the chemically pure substance.

Dietary Sources
Many foods of animal and vegetable origin contain riboflavin. The richest sources are milk and its non-fat products. Other good sources are green vegetables, meat (especially liver), fish and eggs. A proportion of the riboflavin is lost when food is cooked, when exposed to sunlight, or if the water in which the food is cooked is discarded. Milk in bottles exposed to direct sunlight loses some of its riboflavin content.

Human Requirements
Recommended daily dietary allowances for riboflavin in the U.S. are set at 1.7 mg. for men and 1.5 mg. for women. An additional 0.3 mg. is recommended for women during the last two-thirds of pregnancy and an additional 0.5 mg. during lactation. Children have relatively higher needs than adults and 0.6 mg. is the recommended allowance during infancy and this ranges up to 1.5 mg. for adolescent boys.

These allowances provide what is considered a reasonable margin of safety. The minimum requirement to prevent clinical signs of deficiency is believed to be about 0.3 mg. per 1000 calories in adults.

Deficiency
Naturally occurring riboflavin deficiency alone has not been shown to cause serious life threatening disease in man. Ariboflavinosis does however lead to lesions of the lips, mouth, eyes, skin and genitalia.[51]

The most common lesions are angular stomatitis and cheilosis of the lips. Angular stomatitis consists of fissures or cracks radiating from the angles of the mouth onto the skin. Sometimes the lesions extend onto the mucous membrane inside the mouth. These cracks have a raw appearance but may become yel-

51. Keys, A. et al., *J. Nutr.* 26:399, 1943.

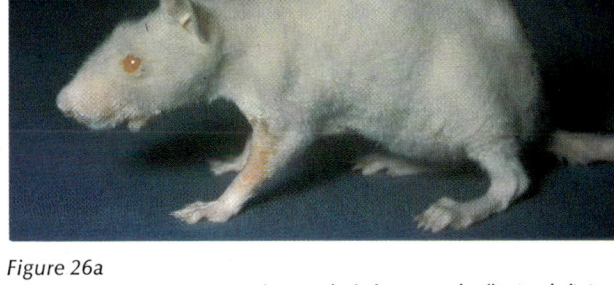

Figure 26a
Generalized dermatitis and growth failure in riboflavin-deficient rat. There is marked keratitis of the cornea.

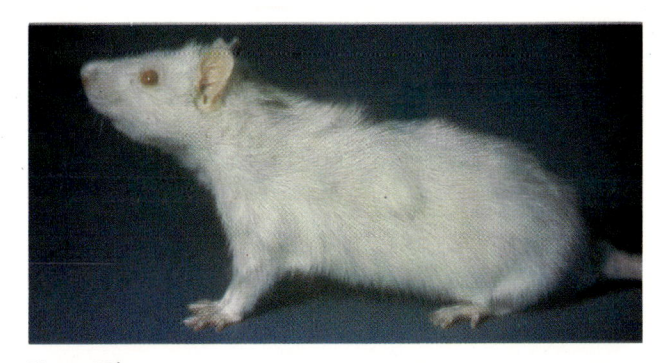

Figure 26b
After one month of treatment with riboflavin the animal shows improvement. Growth has been resumed and ocular and skin lesions are practically gone.

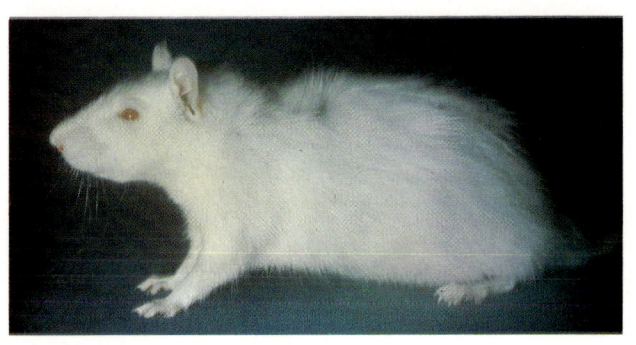

Figure 26c
After two months of treatment the rat shows no signs of the original deficiency.

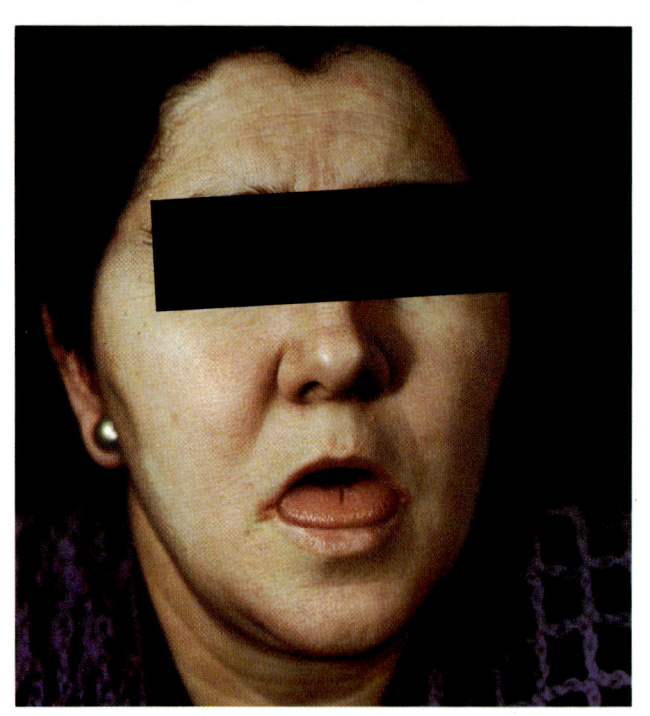

Figure 27a
Riboflavin deficiency manifested as fissures at angle of mouth.

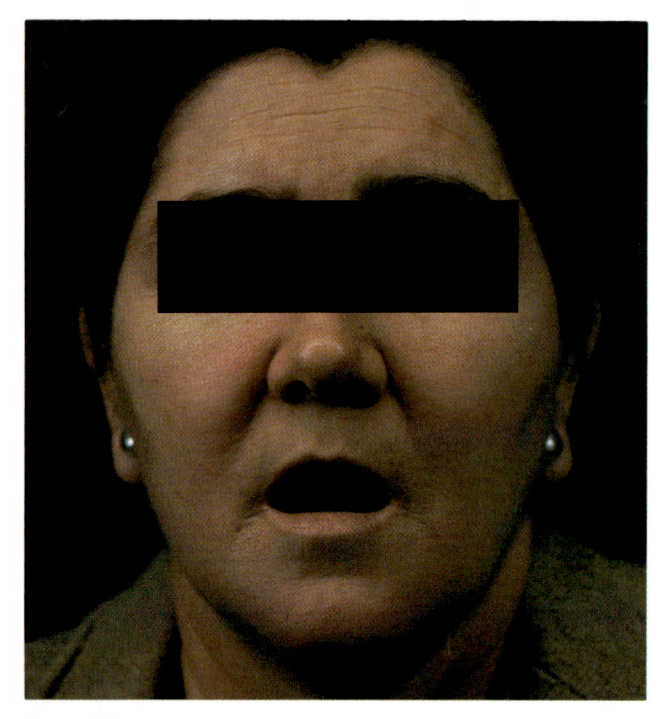

Figure 27b
Complete eradication after treatment with riboflavin therapy.

lowish due to secondary infection. Cheilosis of the lip is a condition in which there are painful cracks on the upper and lower lips. The lips may be swollen and denuded at the line of closure. The lesions may be red and sore, or dry and healing.

Less commonly, glossitis develops and causes a patchy denudation, papillary atrophy and so-called magenta tongue. These latter conditions are not exclusively due to riboflavin deficiency.

In males scrotal dermatitis (vulval dermatitis in females) has been particularly well described in experimental riboflavin deficiency. The affected skin is usually intensely itchy and tends to desquamate. The resulting scratching leads to redness, excoriation and sometimes infection.

Eye lesions, again not specific to riboflavin deficiency, include vascularization of the cornea, photophobia and lacrimation. The condition may cause an annoying irritation of the eyes with a sensation of itching and burning.

Dyssebacea which is most commonly seen in the naso-labial folds but may involve the nose, the canthi of the eyes and occasionally the ears is a feature of riboflavin deficiency and other conditions. If visualized with a magnifying glass the condition is seen as plugs of yellowish colored keratin standing out from the ducts of enlarged sebaceous glands.

Toxicity

Excess intake of riboflavin spills into the urine. Toxicity in man has not been described.

Figure 28

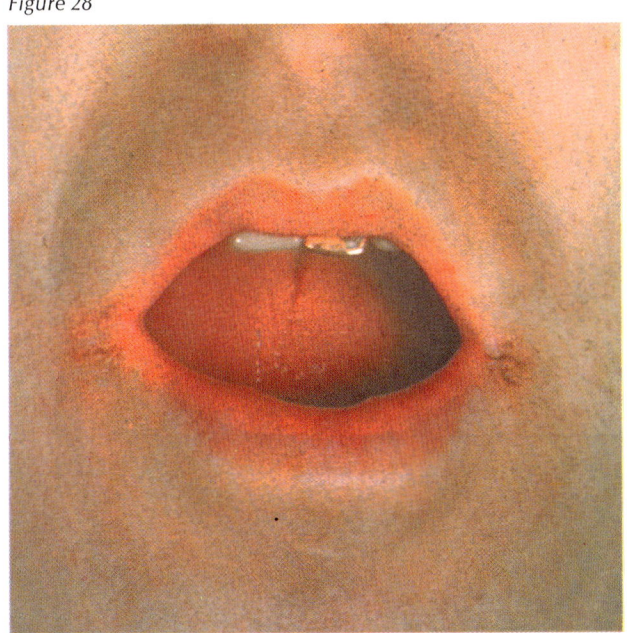

Figure 29

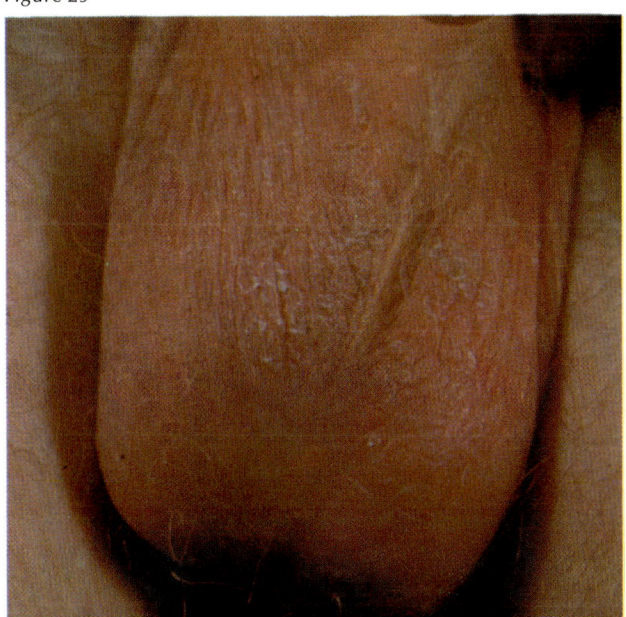

Induced riboflavin deficiency. Twelve of 15 male patients maintained for 9-17 months on a riboflavin-deficient but otherwise adequate diet (0.55 mg. riboflavin daily per 2,200 calories) displayed clinical signs of deficiency including angular stomatitis, seborrheic dermatitis and scaly scrotal skin lesions. Three of the four controls who were on the vitamin-deficient diet supplemented with 2 mg. riboflavin daily, developed scrotal erythema with little or no scaling.

Figure 28
Angular stomatitis with bilateral fissures. Left oral lesion began after about 4½ months on the deficient diet and continued in a fluctuating state of exacerbation and remission for several months. Right lesion appeared 6 weeks after one at left with no preceding infection, and healed in about three weeks without recurrence.

Figure 29
One patient developed scaly pruritic dermatitis on an erythematous base involving only the anterior aspect of the scrotum bilaterally. Other developments in this patient were patchy seborrhea of the scalp, resistant to treatment and vertical fissures around the nostrils following a respiratory infection and progressed to a weeping, crusty lesion. With 6 mg. of riboflavin added to the diet, improvement of the scrotal lesion was prompt and unequivocal; healing of the more chronic lesions was slower but also definite.

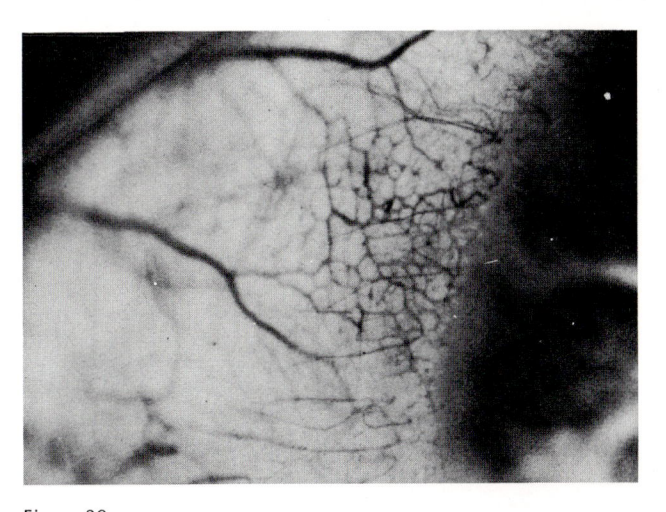

Figure 30
Beginning vascularization of the cornea. Vessels of the limbic plexus have proliferated and invaded the cornea. Vascularization may be accompanied by itching, burning, a feeling of grittiness in the eyes, and photophobia. All symptoms and signs regress after treatment with the vitamin riboflavin.

Figure 31
Skin lesions in pellagra.

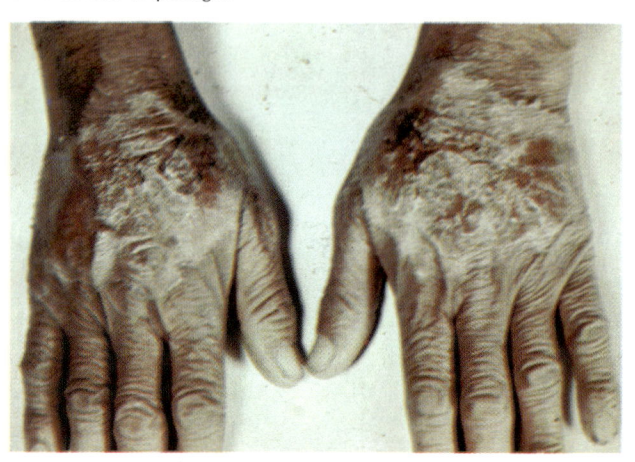

NIACIN (NICOTINIC ACID)

History

Just as the history of thiamine is linked with the disease beriberi so the history of niacin is inextricably woven with the story of the disease pellagra. The association of beriberi is with the Far East and a rice diet, that of pellagra with the New World and with corn (maize) eating peoples.

Well over 200 years ago Casal attributed pellagra to a poor diet and yet it was not until this century that the nutrient responsible was described and isolated. Confusion was caused in part because the disease pellagra could be cured by a protein rich diet and therefore was thought to be due to a protein deficiency. Later a liver extract almost devoid of protein was shown to cure pellagra and in 1926 Goldberger demonstrated that yeast extract contained a pellagra-preventing non-protein substance. In 1937 niacinamide (nicotinc acid amide) was isolated by Elvehjem and this was found to cure "black tongue," a pellagra-like disease which occurred in dogs.

Properties

Niacin functions in the body as a component of two coenzymes important in glycolysis and tissue respiration. It is a simple derivative of pyridine and is extremely stable. Niacin is a water soluble white compound which is moderately resistant to heat and to both acid and alkaline solutions. It is related chemically to nicotine but has very different physiological properties and is essentially non-toxic. It has recently been found that niacin (but not niacinamide) in very large oral doses will lower serum cholesterol (beta-lipoproteins and triglycerides) in man.

Niacin has been accepted in the United States as the name for nicotinic acid, and niacinamide for nicotinic acid amide.

Units

Niacin is measured in milligrams of the synthesized pure substance.

Dietary sources

Niacin is present in many foods of vegetable origin and niacinamide in most foods from animal sources. Particularly rich are lean meat (especially liver), peanuts, yeast and cereal bran or germ. Like other B vitamins the main source in the diet is frequently the cereal staple consumed. Whole grain or lightly milled cereals contain more niacin than refined cereal grains and flours. Niacin is now often added to many manufactured food products especially those made from cereals.

Beans, peas and other legumes are good sources but starchy roots such as potatoes and cassava (manioc, yucca), common vegetables and fruits and milk are all poor sources of the vitamin.

The human body has the ability to convert the amino acid tryptophan to niacin. It is believed that about 60 mg. of dietary tryptophan is equivalent to 1 mg. of niacin. Diets in the U.S. often contain 600 mg. or more of tryptophan and this provides a substantial contribution to the niacin pool. However, diets of poor persons in the U.S. and elsewhere are usually low in protein and in these people pellagra is likely to occur. The tryptophan content of their diets is often as low as 150 mg.

Corn is poor in niacin and its principal protein, zein, is very low in tryptophan content. There is evidence that some of the niacin in corn is present in a bound form and may be unavailable.

Human Requirements

Because niacin is obtained pre-formed or from tryptophan the recommended allowances are stated as niacin equivalents. These include the pre-formed vitamin and the precursor tryptophan (60 mg. tryptophan representing 1 mg. niacin). Allowances for adults in the U.S. are set at 18 mg. for males and 13 mg. for females with a recommendation of an extra 2 mg. during the second and third trimesters of pregnancy and an extra 7 mg. during lactation. Children have proportionately higher requirements and an intake of 5 to 8 mg. is recommended for infants and up to 20 mg. for adolescent boys.

The recommended allowance based on a calorie intake and expressed in niacin equivalents is 6.6 mg. per 1000 calories and not less than 13 mg. if the daily caloric intake is between 1000-2000.

It is believed that the minimum requirement to prevent pellagra averages 4.4 mg./1000 calories per day or a minimum intake in adults of 9.0 mg. per day particularly if the caloric value is less than 2000 calories.

Deficiency

A deficiency of the vitamin leads to the disease pellagra.

Toxicity

Both niacin and niacinamide may be regarded as non-toxic because there is very wide margin between their therapeutic and toxic doses.

Niacin (but not niacinamide) acts as a vasodilator and therefore may cause a flushing of the skin, dizziness and nausea. These symptoms are temporary and in no way harmful. Because of these vasomotor symptoms, niacinamide is preferable to niacin, especially when large doses are needed for the treatment of pellagra. But as previously mentioned, large doses of niacin lower blood cholesterol where niacinamide does not have this effect.

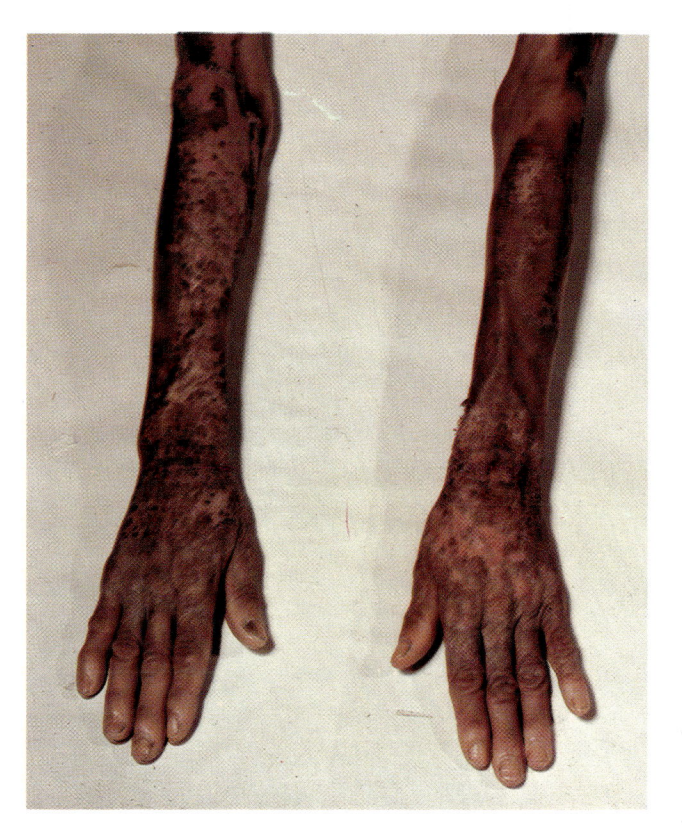

Figure 32a
Pellagrous dermatitis in advanced stage.

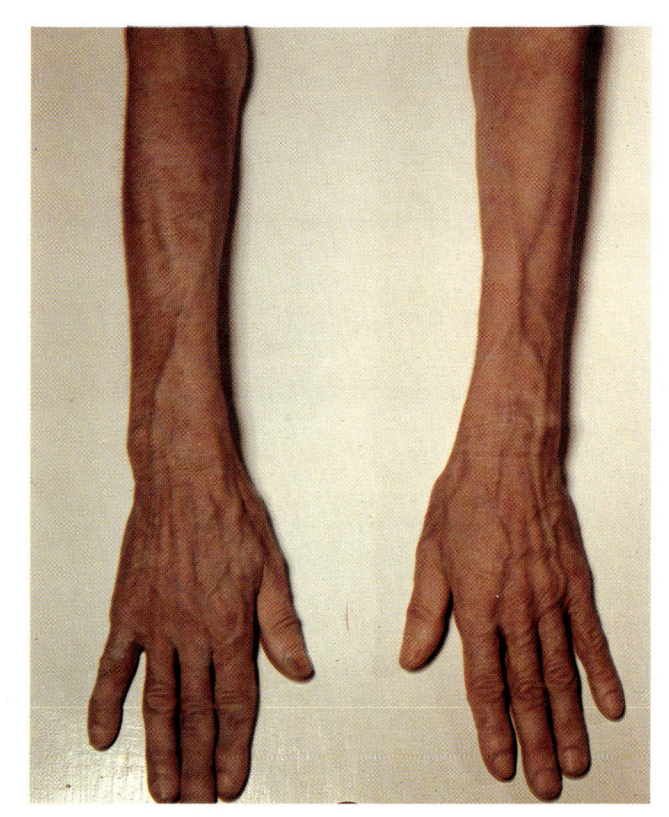

Figure 32b
Same patient after intensive niacin therapy.

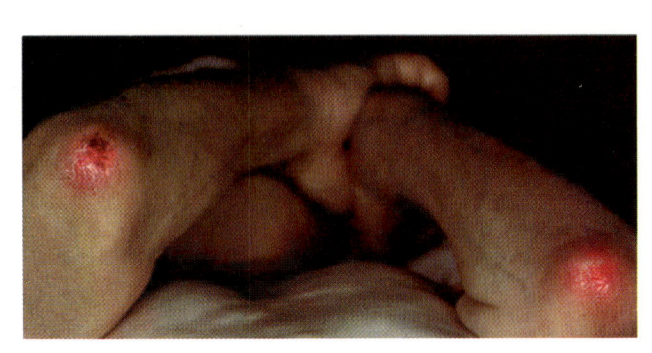

Figure 33
Nicotinamide deficiency–advanced pellagra.
Dermatitis of elbows is precipitated by friction and shows initial desquamation in the center of the lesion. With periods of remission, residual pigmentation persists and becomes deeper with repeated attacks.

VITAMIN B₆

Vitamin B₆ is a useful term because it covers three pyridine derivatives all of which occur in food and which are interconverted metabolically in the human. These substances are pyridoxal and pyridoxamine present mainly in animal products and pyridoxine, present mainly in plants.

Properties

Vitamin B₆ is involved in the metabolism of amino acids and it is an essential part of the enzyme glycogen phosphorylase.

Units

The activity of pyridoxine is expressed in milligrams of the synthesized pure substance.

Sources

Vitamin B₆ is widely distributed in foods of both animal and vegetable origin. Whole grain cereals, milk, meat (especially liver and kidney) and certain vegetables are good sources of the vitamin which is easily absorbed.

Requirements

A recommended daily dietary allowance was first set for this vitamin in 1968. The recommended allowance for adults is 2 milligrams daily plus an additional 0.5 milligram daily during pregnancy and lactation.

Deficiency

Vitamin B₆ deficiency tends to increase the oxalate excretion in the urine. A vitamin deficiency involving vesical stone formation[52] may occur in certain areas of the world where these are common, e.g., Thailand. Some success in treating renal calcium oxalate calculi with magnesium oxide and vitamin B₆ has been reported.

Vitamin B₆ deficiency in infants manifests itself by hyperirritability, convulsions and anemia. An inborn error of metabolism leading to a dependency on a high intake of vitamin B₆ has been described. It is seen during the first seven days of life and leads to convulsions. Unless treated early with vitamin B₆ the child may become mentally retarded. Vitamin B₆ responsive anemias have been reported in adults.

Increasingly important in clinical medicine is the B₆ deficiency which follows treatment of tuberculosis with isonicotinic and acid hydrazide (isoniazid or INH).[53] This drug apparently leads to increased requirements for vitamin B₆ by interfering with certain activities of pyridoxal phosphate. Patients on a poor diet taking INH may develop a severe polyneuritis which may be both painful and disabling. Administration of pyridoxine in daily doses of 10-20 mg. per day may be useful in preventing this complication of tuberculosis treatment.

There is some evidence that pregnant women develop a deficiency and that vitamin B₆ supplementation may be of value in treating the nausea of pregnancy.

Adequacy of vitamin B₆ nutriture is often assessed by measuring the urinary excretion of tryptophan metabolites, particularly xanthurenic acid following a tryptophan load test.

52. Gershoff, S. N. et al., *Am. J. Clin. Nutr. 8*:812, 1960.
53. Biehl, J. P. and Vilter, R. W., *JAMA 156*:549, 1954.

Figure 34
Oxalate bladder stones in Thailand.

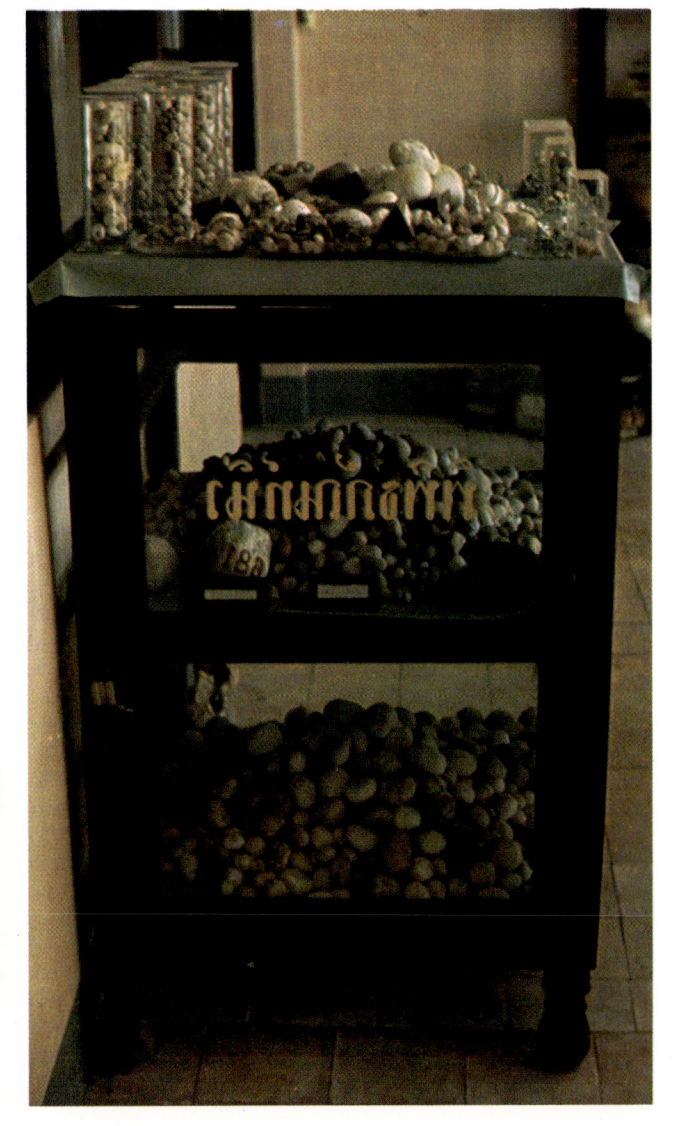

Treatment of convulsions in pyridoxine-deficient infant.

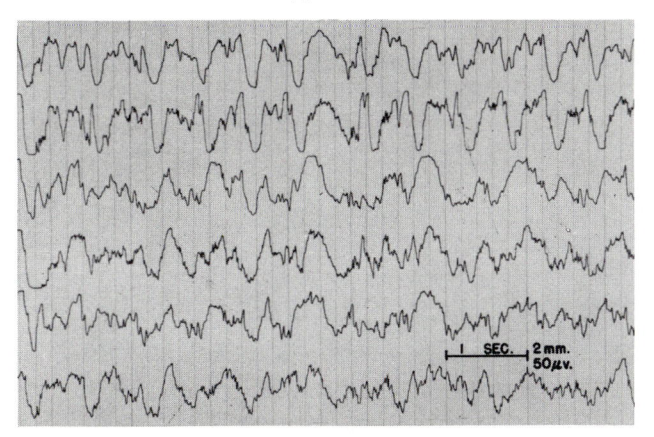

Figure 35a
Electroencephalogram of infant during convulsions produced by pyridoxine deficiency.

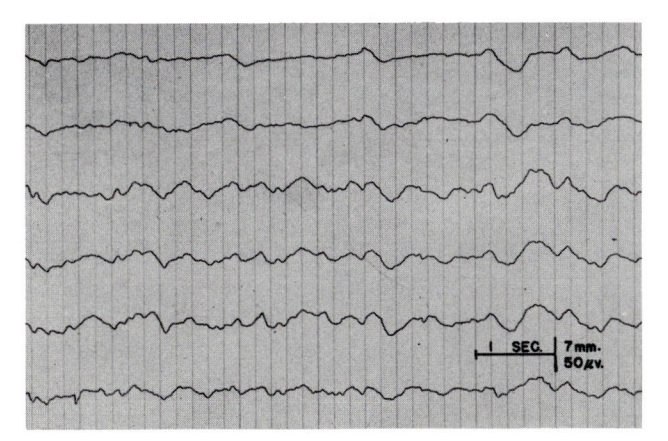

Figure 35b
Five minutes after pyridoxine administration; color improved and the infant slept.

Experimentally induced B_6 deficiency leads to loss of appetite and weight, general weakness and lassitude and certain symptoms and signs normally ascribed to deficiencies of other B vitamins. These include cheilosis, glossitis, peripheral neuritis and skin changes reminiscent of pellagra.

Toxicity
Toxicity to vitamin B_6 has been described in men receiving 300 mg./day, a dose far in excess of any therapy recommended for drug treatment and a dose impossible to receive from foods.

PANTOTHENIC ACID

Properties

Pantothenic acid is a part of coenzyme A and is involved in the release of energy from carbohydrate. It is vital to the synthesis and degradation of sterols, fatty acids and steroid hormones. Pantothenic acid is also involved in the acetylation of choline.

Units

The activity of pantothenic acid is expressed in milligrams of the synthesized pure substance.

Dietary Sources

Pantothenic acid is widely distributed and freely available in ordinary foods so that a deficiency is rare in humans receiving a natural or even a marginally adequate diet.

Deficiency

Various studies on volunteers on a diet deficient in pantothenic acid and with a pantothenic acid antagonist, omega methyl pantothenic acid, develop tiredness, abdominal pain and cramps, nausea, sometimes flatulence and vomiting and paresthesia of the hands and feet.[54]

The "burning feet" syndrome accompanied by severe parathesia and great tenderness of the feet in prisoners-of-war on very poor diets in World War II was believed to be in part due to pantothenic acid deficiency.

Human Requirements

Probably 10 mg. of pantothenic acid daily will satisfy human requirements. Most diets in the U.S. contain around 15 mg. per day, even low cost diets.

Toxicity

Toxicity is not known to occur in man.

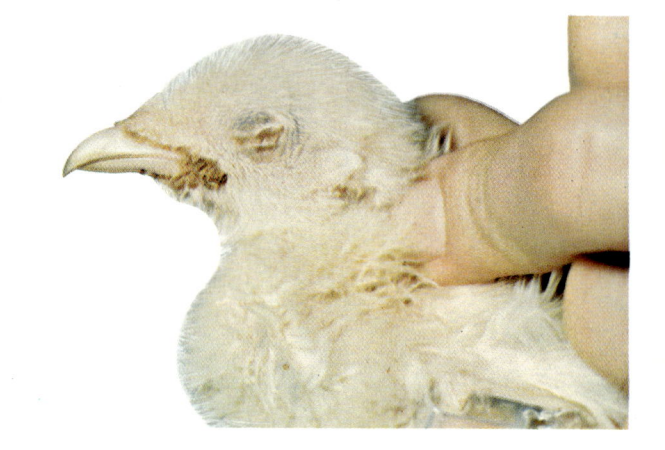

Figure 36a
Dermatitis in a chick whose diet was deficient in pantothenic acid. The eyelids, corners of the mouth, and adjacent skin are involved. Feathering is retarded and rough.

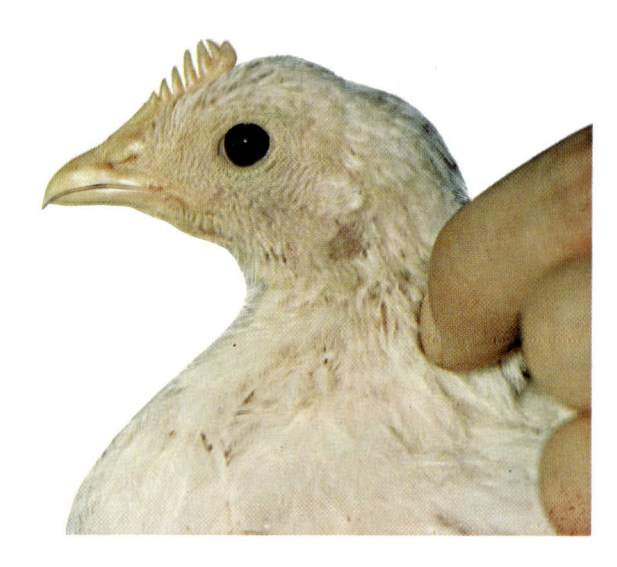

Figure 36b
Three weeks after calcium pantothenate was added to the diet, skin lesions were cured.

54. Hodges, R. E. et al., *J. Clin. Invest.* 38:1421, 1959.

CYANOCOBALAMIN (B₁₂)

History

The disease pernicious anemia, so named because it was invariably fatal, was described in detail by Addison in England in 1849. About 40 years ago it was found by Minot and Murphy that the disease improved if the patient consumed raw liver. Soon after this Castle showed that beef mixed with normal gastric juice caused remission in subjects with pernicious anemia but that neither component alone was effective. Castle called the factor in the meat "extrinsic factor." He suggested that the two together interact to produce a substance present in raw liver which relieves pernicious anemia.

It was not until 1948 that the anti-PA vitamin of liver extract was finally isolated independently in England and in the U.S.A. Within a very short time cyanocobalamin (vitamin B_{12}) was shown to improve the hematological picture of pernicious anemia as well as to prevent the neurological complication of subacute degeneration of the spinal cord.

Properties

Cyanocobalamin (vitamin B_{12}) is a red crystalline cobalt-containing substance which is soluble in water and is resistent to heat. It is readily destroyed by strong acids and alkalis, and also by sunlight. Cyanocobalamin consists of a heavy complex non-protein molecule. In food it is bound to protein and it is now believed that the intrinsic factor, an enzyme secreted by the stomach, removes the B_{12} from its protein combination. It is then absorbed from the small intestine and is stored in the liver and to a lesser extent in the kidney.

Cyanocobalamin is essential for the function of all cells but particularly for cells of the bone marrow, the intestinal tract and the central nervous system. Being active in very small amounts it is an extremely potent catalyst and appears to facilitate reduction reactions such as the conversion of ribose to deoxyribose and of formyl through methyl reduction to tetrahydrofolic

Bone marrow smears in pernicious anemia before and after vitamin B_{12} therapy.

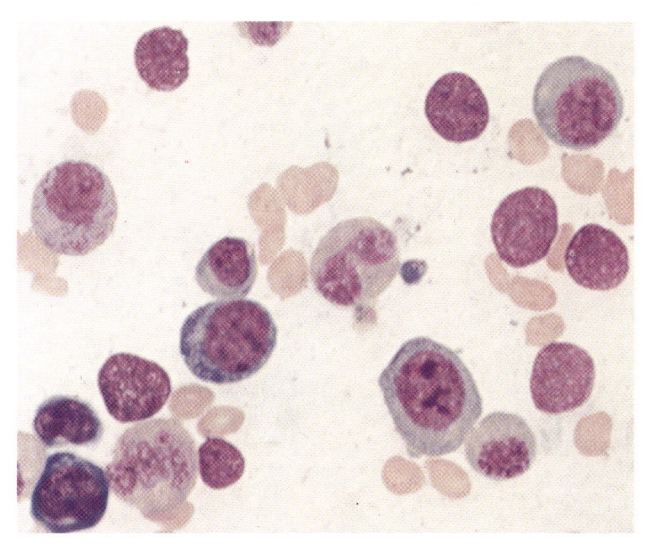

Figure 37a
Smear showing a number of megaloblasts, characteristic of certain anemias.

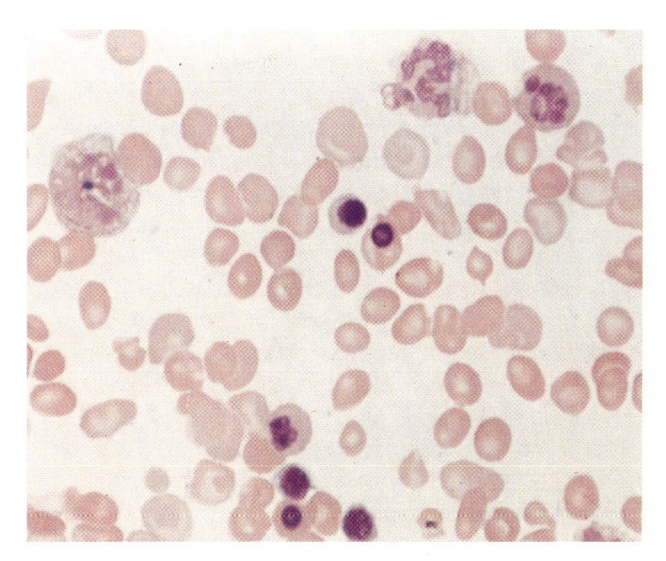

Figure 37b
Within 48-72 hours after treatment with 25 micrograms of vitamin B_{12} the megaloblasts have been replaced by normoblasts.

acid.[55] It also acts as a cofactor in the transfer of a methyl group to homocysteine to form methionine. It is probably involved in the metabolism of protein, carbohydrate and fat but it is of greatest importance in nucleic acid and folic acid metabolic processes.

Units

Activity of cyanocobalamin is expressed in milligrams and micrograms of the pure crystalline substance.

Dietary Sources

Cyanocobalamin is obtained in human diets from foods of animal origin, particularly meat (liver and kidney are very rich) and dairy products. Negligible quantities are present in foods of vegetable origin. Herbivores obtain their cyanocobalamin from bacterial synthesis in the rumen, but in man intestinal microbial synthesis provides very little of the vitamin.

Cyanocobalamin occurring in food is poorly absorbed in the absence of intrinsic factor. Storage of vitamin B_{12} in the human is good.

Human Requirements

In normal adults a diet containing 5 micrograms of cyanocobalamin daily will satisfy requirements. Diets in the U.S. show marked variation in their content of B_{12}. This is because meat, fish and other animal products are relatively expensive and as a result there are wide class differences in the quantities consumed. High cost diets contain about 31 micrograms and low cost diets as little as 2.7 micrograms of vitamin B_{12}. Absorption is inversely related to the intake of the vitamin in a range from 30 to 70 percent.

Persons with pernicious anemia or with megaloblastic anemia due to dietary lack of cyanocobalamin often respond to as little as 0.1 microgram of the vitamin given by injection.[56] Normally 0.5-2.0 micrograms given daily parenterally will maintain complete remission, but doses of 2-4 micrograms are needed to replenish liver stores. Once saturation has occurred about 1.5 micrograms of cyanocobalamin daily will maintain and satisfy the biochemical needs of the body. Recommended daily dietary allowances are 5 micrograms for adults, 6 micrograms for the elderly, and 8 micrograms during pregnancy.

Deficiency

Pernicious anemia is a manifestation of vitamin B_{12} deficiency but is not due to a straight forward dietary deficiency of the vitamin. There is a defect, probably genetic, which results in impaired secretion of intrinsic factor by the stomach. A constant finding in pernicious anemia is absence or reduced amounts of both intrinsic factor and free HCl in the gastric juice. Pernicious anemia leads to weakness, to oral manifestations and to signs of central nervous system involvement. A soreness of the tongue is often intermittent but when present the tongue is red and inflamed looking and between attacks there is evidence of papillary atrophy. The tongue eventually becomes smooth and glazed. Concomitant with the glossitis are lesions of other mucous surfaces of the mouth including the lips. The neurologic manifestations are indicative of lesions in both the lateral and posterior spinal cord with peripheral nerve degeneration. Pallor, palpitations and eventually more severe cardiovascular disturbances are all features of the anemia.

Gastrectomy if fairly radical may cause a similar condition because the secreting cells of the stomach are removed.

Persons who live exclusively on vegetable products and who do not even eat dairy products and eggs are called vegans or "strict" vegetarians. Most vegetarians commonly consume milk and its by-products and also eggs and are really "lacto-ovo-vegetarians." Vegans are likely to develop most of the signs of pernicious anemia including glossitis and evidence of involvement of the long tracts of the spinal cord but do not usually develop anemia.[57]

55. Cantarow, A. and Schepartz, B., *Biochemistry,* 3rd Edition, W. B. Saunders Company, Philadelphia, 1962.
56. Sullivan, W. and Herbert, V., *Am. J. Clin. Nutr.* 10:354, 1962.
57. Wokes, F., Badenock, J., and Sinclair, H. M., *Am. J. Clin. Nutr.* 3:375, 1955.

Figure 38
The tongue in pernicious anemia is typically pale and shiny, the papillae having atrophied in the course of the glossitis which is often the first symptom of the disease. The tongue may become red and sore; these symptoms usually subside promptly with therapy, but may recur in a relapse. Adequate therapy restores the tongue's normal color and may partially restore the papillae.

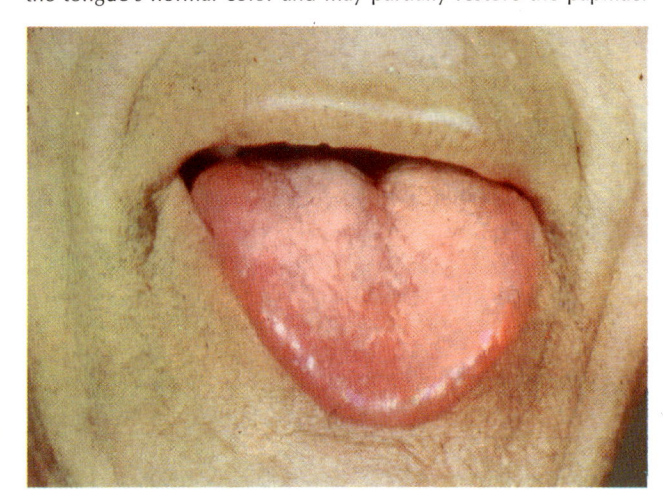

Diphyllobothrium latum, the fish tapeworm, has a propensity for removing cyanocobalamin from the food in the intestine of its host. This may result in megaloblastic anemia which can be cured by injection of the vitamin.

Cyanocobalamin deficiency complicated by a deficiency of folic acid and other nutrients is a feature of sprue and other malabsorption syndromes.

Toxicity
Cyanocobalamin is not toxic to man when given by mouth or injection in amounts very much larger than those recommended for therapeutic purposes.

FOLACIN (Folic acid, folate and pteroylglutamic acid)
History
In the early 1930's, Dr. Lucy Wills, in India, clearly indicated the public health importance of megaloblastic anemia in pregnant women. She also demonstrated good clinical response to some antianemic principle in autolysed yeast. This principle was ineffective in Addisonian pernicious anemia and was different from cyanocobalamin present in liver extract. In 1941 Mitchell and his colleagues in the U.S. obtained from spinach leaves a substance they called folic acid which was important in the growth of certain microorganisms. A few years later folic acid was synthesized and shown to have a beneficial hemopoietic effect in pernicious anemia. The immediate high hopes were lessened when it was found that folic acid did not prevent the neurological lesions of this disease.

Properties
Folic acid is a yellow substance which is slightly soluble in water. The function of folacin coenzymes is the transfer of single carbon units in intracellular synthesis, particularly of purine and serine.[58,59,60] Folacin is stored mainly in the liver. Blood, serum and urine contain folacin in many different forms and these act as growth factors for certain non-pathogenic bacteria normally present in the human thus complicating physiologic studies of the vitamin.

There has been much research on the precise role of folacin in hemopoiesis. Most evidence suggests that folate deficiency anemia is extremely difficult to produce in mammals unless a folic acid antagonist is administered or certain conditions exist concurrent with the folate deficiency. These include ascorbic acid deficiency, a bacteria-free intestinal tract or a high level of methionine added to the diet.

Units
Folacin activity is reported as milligrams and micrograms of the crystalline pure substance.

Dietary Sources
Dark green edible leaves, kidney, liver, and vegetables are the richest sources of the vitamin in human diets. Smaller amounts are present in meat, cereals, fruits and some roots. Milk, eggs and poultry are poor sources. Storage of food and particularly cooking cause considerable vitamin loss. The vitamin is readily absorbed from the normal intestine.

58. Luhby, A. L. et al., *Advances Metab. Dis.* 1:263, 1964.
59. Herbert, V., *Am. J. Clin. Nutr.* 20:562, 1967.
60. Vilter, R. W. et al., *Am. J. Clin. Nutr.* 12:130, 1963.

Human Requirements

Recommended daily dietary allowances were first set by the Food and Nutrition Board in 1968. The recommendation is 0.4 milligrams of folacin for adults with an additional 0.1 milligram during lactation and an additional 0.4 milligram during pregnancy.

Deficiency

Macrocytic anemia is the main manifestation of folic acid deficiency in the human. It is characterized by lesions of the alimentary tract including stomatitis, glossitis, changes in the intestines, diarrhea and malabsorption.

Megaloblastic anemia of pregnancy occurs because of the increased needs for the vitamin during pregnancy, vomiting which is sometimes persistent during pregnancy, the dietary lack of the vitamin in the diets of some pregnant women and possibly because of a metabolic defect in the production of the folic acid coenzymes.

In sprue and other malabsorption syndromes there is a folate deficiency because of impaired absorption and often megaloblastic anemia is present. This may also be accompanied by vitamin B_{12} deficiency.

A nutritional macrocytic anemia may occur in subjects on an exceedingly poor diet. Megaloblastic anemia may result from a combination of folic acid and vitamin C deficiency in persons with scurvy. Infants on a diet purely of milk may also develop a nutritional macrocytic anemia, as milk is deficient in both folic acid and ascorbic acid.

Megaloblastic anemia in alcoholics may be due to their generally poor dietary habits and is usually associated with low folate intakes. It has been suggested that iron deficiency may also result in a functional defect in folate utilization.

Herbert in 1962 reported on experimental folate deficiency, placing himself on a low folate diet. In four months he developed megaloblastic anemia and other signs of folacin deficiency.[61]

61. Herbert, V., *Tr. Assoc. Am. Phys.* 75:307, 1962.

Perhaps no other nutrient has caused so much debate or confusion as has folacin in causing a dietary deficiency disease in man. It is not absolutely clear whether the deficiency causes or is caused by morphological changes in the intestinal tract. The answer is probably that folacin deficiency induced by some extraneous cause is a more important public health problem than is a true dietary folacin deficiency.

Toxicity

Folacin is not toxic to the normal human even in doses much larger than those usually consumed or even those used as a therapeutic measure. The dangers of doses above 0.1 mg. per day is that they may prevent the neurologic manifestations of this disease. In the United States at the present time it is illegal to sell without a prescription vitamin preparations recommending doses of more than 0.1 mg. folic acid daily.[62] Physicians prescribing folic acid should be aware of this potential danger.

VITAMIN C (ASCORBIC ACID)

History

The history of vitamin C is linked with that of scurvy. This disease was known long before the vitamin era as several centuries ago the anti-scorbutic effects of certain foods were described. In those early days scurvy was a particular scourge of sailors taking voyages of many weeks without fresh food. It was however not until 1747 that James Lind of Scotland demonstrated that scurvy could be cured or prevented by the consumption of citrus fruit. This led, well before the discovery of vitamins, to the inclusion of certain fresh foods and fruits in sailors' diets.

In the 19th century, scurvy began to occur for the first time among infants when they were being fed with the newly introduced powdered and canned

62. *Recommended Dietary Allowances*, 7th Edition, NAS-NRC, Publication 1694, Washington, D.C., 1968.

Megaloblastic anemia of pregnancy treated with folic acid. Patient, 32, hospitalized with severe anemia two weeks after delivery of her fifth child, responded within 48 hours to intravenous folic acid therapy.

Chart 9

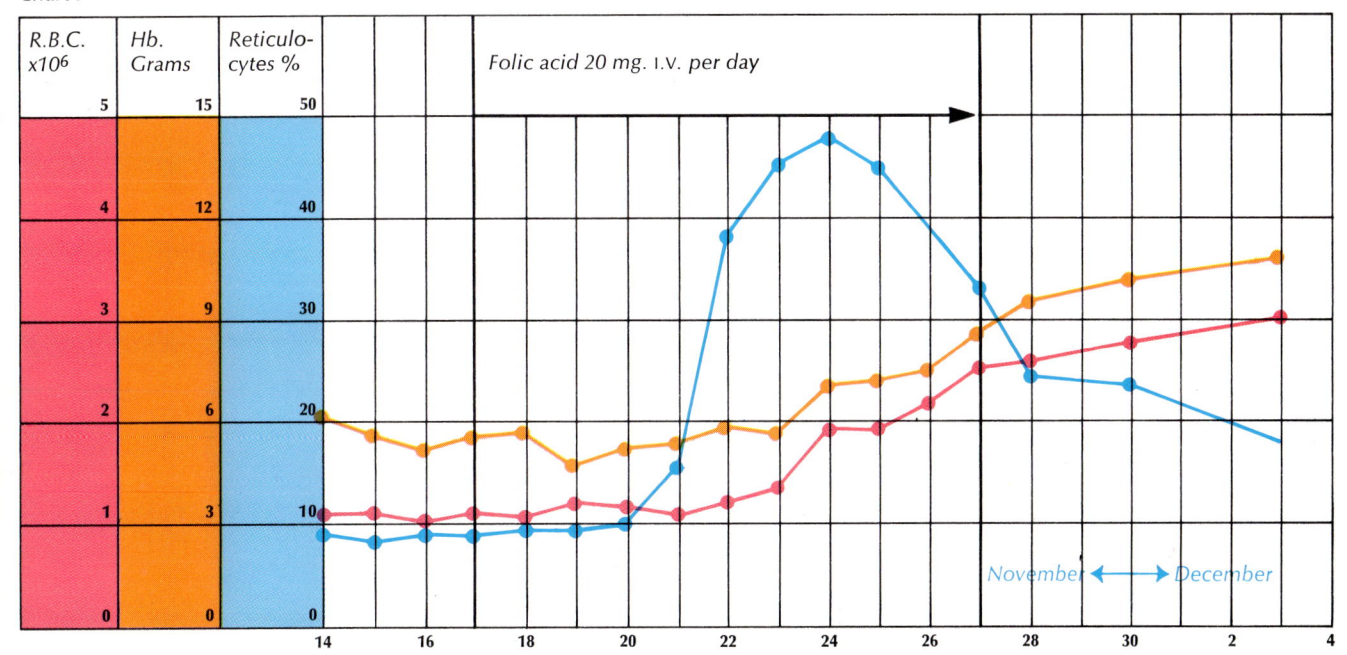

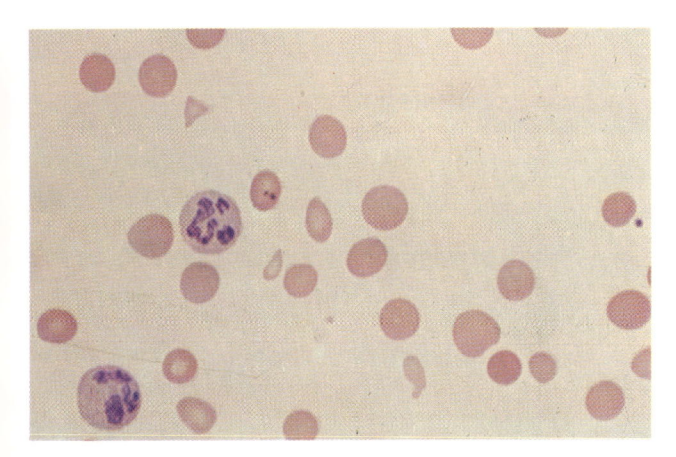

Figure 39a
Inset of peripheral blood illustrates the characteristic poikilocytosis and anisocytosis of untreated macrocytic anemia.

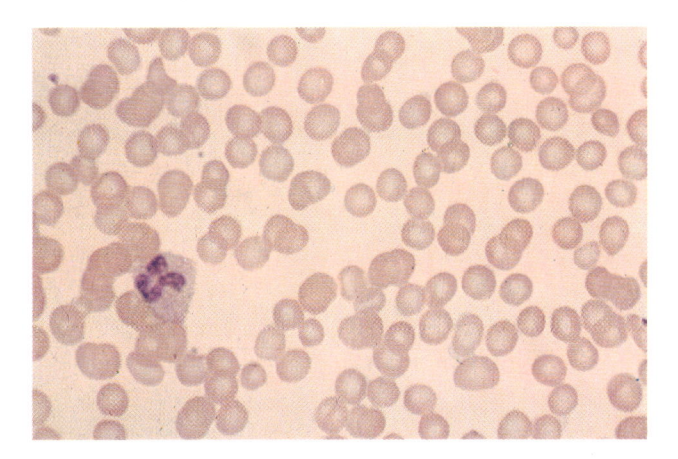

Figure 39b
Illustrates the recovery of the red cells' normal size and shape after therapy. Polymorphonuclear leukocytes, included in the photographs to indicate comparative cell size, also show, prior to treatment, the hypersegmentation typical of macrocytic anemias.

81

milks instead of the usual diet of breast milk or fresh cows' milk. The vitamin C had been destroyed when these milk products were heated during preparation.

In spite of the value attributed to vitamin C, ascorbic acid wasn't isolated until 1928 and was finally synthesized in 1932.

Properties

Ascorbic acid is a white crystalline substance very highly soluble in water and readily oxidized. It is not affected by light but is destroyed by excessive heat especially in an alkaline solution.

Vitamin C has many functions in the body. The Recommended Dietary Allowances[63] of the Food and Nutrition Board summarizes ascorbic acid's role in the following metabolic systems:
- a) oxidation of phenylalanine and tyrosine via para-hydroxyphenylpyruvate;
- b) hydroxylation of aromatic compounds;
- c) conversion of folacin to folinic acid;
- d) regulation of the respiratory cycle in mitochondria and microsomes;
- e) hydrolysis of alkyl monothioglycosides;
- f) development of odontoblasts and other specialized cells including collagen and cartilage and
- g) maintaining the mechanical strength of blood vessels particularly the venules.

It is the failure of this latter function which leads to several of the signs and symptoms of scurvy including hemorrhage into various tissues.

Units

Ascorbic acid is measured in milligrams and grams. In some textbooks it is still referred to in terms of International Units. The original I.U. was defined as the amount of vitamin C present in 0.1 ml. of lemon juice.

Dietary Sources

Vitamin C is less widely present in foodstuffs than are the other important water-soluble vitamins. In

63. *Recommended Dietary Allowances,* 7th Edition, NAS-NRC, Publication 1694, Washington, D.C.,1968.

Figure 40
Gingival lesions in advanced scurvy.

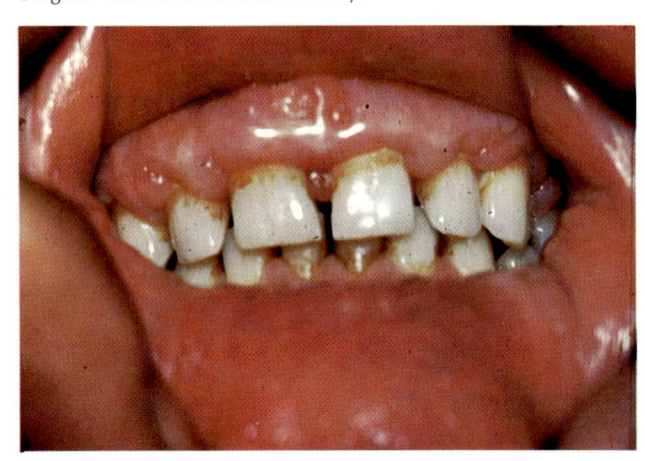

normal United States diets the main source is from citrus fruits, juices, tomatoes and other fruits and vegetables. Eggs, meat and fish are rather poor sources, as is milk after pasteurization. Dried cereal grains and the seeds of legumes are devoid of vitamin C unless sprouting. Vitamin C is often added to many beverages and some foods and if so, the label will so indicate.

Human Requirements

The daily dietary allowances recommended by the Food and Nutrition Board are 60 mg. for adult males and 55 mg. for females with a recommendation of an additional 5 mg. daily during lactation and pregnancy. Recommended allowances during childhood range from 35 mg. during infancy to 55 mg. during adolescence.

These recommendations almost certainly provide a wide margin of safety and in our opinion ascorbic acid intakes of about two-thirds of the recommended allowances are more than adequate. It should be noted that in Britian the recommended allowance for vitamin C in adults is 20 mg. and in Canada, Australia, and Norway it is 30 mg.

The difference of opinion is because there are two schools of thought. Those favoring the higher recommendations believe that it is desirable for the body to

Figure 41
In scorbutic rosary, the enlarged costochondral junctions of scurvy resemble those of rickets. The lesions in scurvy may feel sharper and may be somewhat tender.

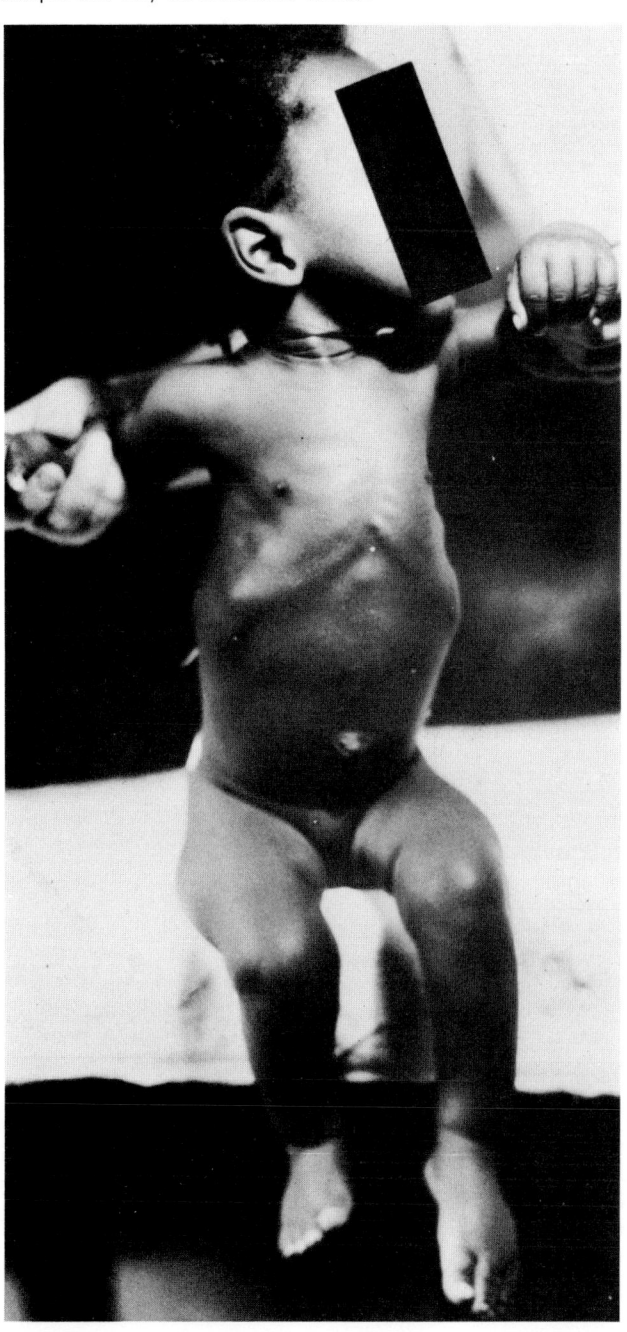

be saturated with the vitamin and those favoring the smaller allowance suggest that the amount should be based on that required to maintain good health. There is no evidence that scurvy or poor healing of wounds or any other abnormality occurs on intakes of 20 mg. daily.

Deficiency

A deficiency of vitamin C leads to the disease scurvy. (See page 43.) There is some evidence that a subclinical deficiency of the vitamin, not sufficient to cause any of the signs of scurvy, may result in slow healing of wounds or ulcers. Therefore persons undergoing surgery, or following trauma or with persistent ulcers, who are suspected of having a low intake of vitamin C, should have a vitamin C-rich-diet or receive supplemental ascorbic acid tablets.

Claims have been made for the efficacy of large doses of ascorbic acid in preventing the common cold. Controlled trials have shown that the vitamin has no benefit in this regard.

Toxicity

Very high doses of ascorbic acid can be taken without the development of any toxic effects. After saturation is reached the body merely excretes the vitamin in the urine.

VITAMIN D

History

It had been postulated that rickets was a nutritional deficiency disease and for many years prior to any knowledge of the vitamin, cod-liver oil had been successfully used in its treatment. It was not until 1919 that a British scientist, Sir Edward Mellanby, using puppies, demonstrated conclusively that the disease was of nutritional origin and that it responded to a vitamin present in cod-liver oil. This led to some confusion because it was already known that cod-liver oil contained vitamin A. In 1922 McCollum isolated a second fat-soluble vitamin from cod-liver oil and called it vitamin D. Around the same time work had

Impaired wound healing.

The first satisfactory controlled experiment in human scurvy was conducted when J.H. Crandon placed himself on an ascorbic acid free diet, supplemented by all other known vitamins, for six months. After three months on the diet, when the ascorbic acid level in the blood had been zero for 44 days, a wound was made in the midback region.

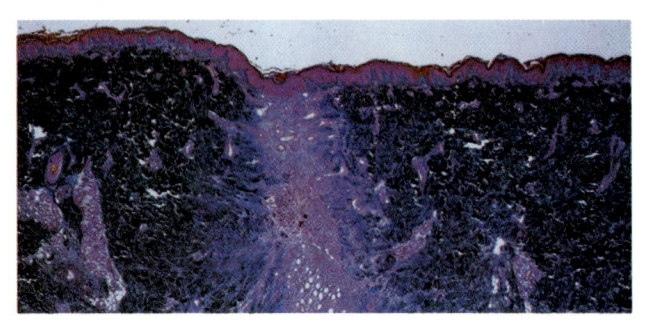

Figure 42a
Biopsy 10 days after this wound shows healing that clinically and pathologically appeared normal, but comparison with Fig. 42c indicates that it was probably suboptimal.

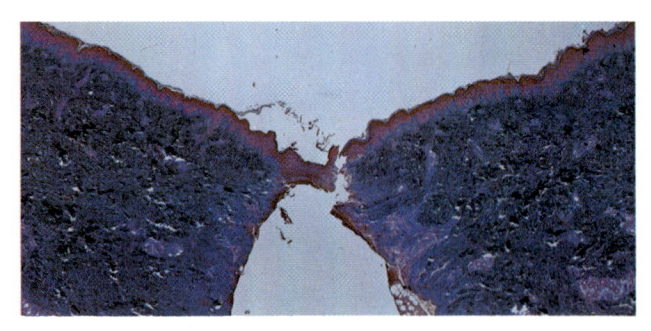

Figure 42b
After six months of the scorbutic diet another wound was made. Biopsy 10 days after second wound shows no healing except of the epithelium (gap in tissues was filled with a blood clot).

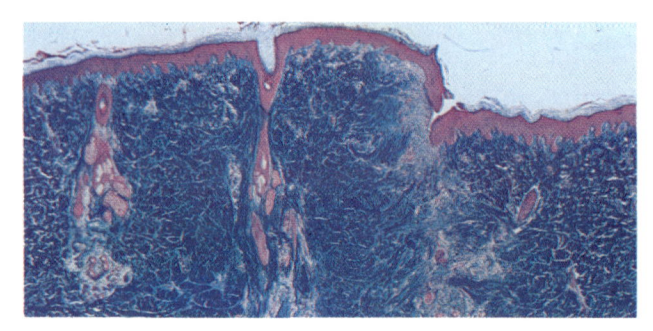

Figure 42c
After 10 days of ascorbic acid treatment another biopsy of the second wound shows healing with abundant collagen formation –considerably more than occurred in the first wound.

been proceeding which led to an explanation of how ultraviolet rays prevented rickets.

Properties

A number of compounds, all sterols, possess anti-rachitic properties. Certain sterols which do not possess anti-rachitic properties become anti-rachitic when exposed to ultraviolet light. The two important activated sterols are vitamin D_2 (activated ergocalciferol) which is derived from plants and vitamin D_3 (activated cholecalciferol) which is found in animal tissues.

In human beings when the skin is exposed to sunlight, a sterol compound (7-dehydrocholesterol) is activated to form vitamin D_3 which then becomes available to the body. This activity is identical to vitamin D ingested in the diet. The latter is only absorbed from the gut in the presence of bile.

Vitamin D promotes the absorption of calcium from the gut and is essential to the maintenance of calcium and phosphorus homeostasis, and to the formation of sound teeth and bones.

Units

Vitamin D is measured in International Units. One I.U. is equivalent to the activity of 0.025 μg. of crystalline vitamin D_2 (ergocalciferol) or 0.025 μg. of pure vitamin D_3 (cholecalciferol).

Dietary Sources

Vitamin D occurs naturally only in the fat of certain food products of animal origin. Eggs, cheese, milk, and butter are fairly good sources. Meat and fish contribute small quantities. Fish liver oils are very rich in vitamin D (and vitamin A) but the amounts vary. In the U.S. milk is frequently fortified with vitamin D and many other food products, especially those frequently eaten by children, have vitamin D added. The fortification of these basic foods is a very desirable public health procedure.

Human Requirements

The U.S. recommended daily dietary allowance is 10 μg. (400 I.U.) of vitamin D during childhood and

FATS AND OILS

Butter	1 pat	7	16	50	Trace	6	3	2	Trace	1	230	.12	.18	1.3	0
Margarine	1 pat	7	16	50	Trace	6	1	3	1	1	230	—	—	—	0
Cooking Fats:															
Lard	1 Tbsp	14	0	126	0	14	5	6	1	0	0	0	0	0	0
Vegetable fats	1 Tbsp	13	0	106	0	12	3	8	1	0	—	0	0	0	0
Salad Dressings:															
Commercial, mayonnaise type	1 Tbsp	15	41	65	Trace	6	1	1	3	2	33	Trace	Trace	Trace	—
French	1 Tbsp	15	39	72	Trace	7	1	1	3	2	—	—	—	—	—
Mayonnaise	1 Tbsp	15	15	93	Trace	11	2	3	6	Trace	36	Trace	.01	Trace	—
Salad or Cooking Oils:															
Corn	1 Tbsp	14	0	125	0	14	1	4	7	0	—	0	0	0	0
Cottonseed	1 Tbsp	14	0	125	0	14	4	3	7	0	—	0	0	0	0
Olive	1 Tbsp	14	0	125	0	14	2	11	1	0	—	0	0	0	0
Safflower	1 Tbsp	14	0	125	0	14	1	2	10	0	—	0	0	0	0
Soybean	1 Tbsp	14	0	125	0	14	2	3	7	0	—	0	0	0	0

SUGARS AND SWEETS

Chocolate, plain	1 oz	28	1	147	2	9	5	4	Trace	65	77	.02	.10	.1	Trace
Honey	1 Tbsp	21	17	64	Trace	0	0	0	0	1	0	Trace	.01	.1	Trace
Jams, jellies, preserves	1 Tbsp	20	29	55	Trace	Trace	—	—	—	4	Trace	Trace	.01	Trace	1
Syrup	1 Tbsp	20	24	58	0	0	0	0	0	9	0	0	0	0	0
Sugar	1 Tbsp	12	Trace	46	0	0	0	0	0	0	0	0	0	0	0

MISCELLANEOUS ITEMS

Beer (3.6% alcohol)	1 bottle	340	92	171	2	0	0	0	0	15	0	Trace	.11	.8	0
Carbonated beverage	8 oz	240	90	90	0	0	0	0	0	—	0	0	0	0	0
Nuts:															
Peanuts, roasted	1 oz	28	2	160	8	13	3	6	4	10	—	.07	.04	5.4	0
Peanut butter	1 Tbsp	16	2	87	4	7	1	4	2	9	—	.02	.02	2.4	0
Pizza (cheese)	1 (5½" pc.)	75	45	184	7	5	2	3	Trace	117	303	.05	.13	.8	5
Popcorn with margarine	1 cup	28	3	155	2	12	3	7	2	5	462	—	.02	.3	0
Soups, canned:															
Noodle type	1 cup	250	93	68	4	2	Trace	1	1	10	113	.03	.05	1.0	Trace
Tomato	1 cup	245	90	88	2	3	—	—	—	15	1,005	.05	.05	1.2	12

(1) Prepared from "Table of Food Values," Harvard Nutrition Service, Department of Nutrition, 665 Huntington Avenue, Boston, Mass. 02115
* Values rounded

APPENDIX C

APPROXIMATE CHOLESTEROL CONTENT OF SELECTED FOODS
(Values from National Diet-Heart Study, 1965)

Item	Portion	Size (gm.)	Cholesterol per Edible Portion (mg.)
Beef, cooked, trimmed	4 oz.	113	102
cooked, untrimmed	4 oz.	113	113
Brains, cooked, no fat added	3 oz.	85	2674
Butter	1 pat	7	20
Cheese: Cheddar and Processed	1 oz.	28	45
Cottage, Creamed	1 cup	225	23
Cream	1 oz.	28	36
Spreads and Cheese Foods	1 oz.	28	39
Chicken, Turkey, cooked	4 oz.	113	85
Cream: Light (20% fat)	1 tbsp.	15	11
Half and Half (12% fat)	1 tbsp.	15	6
Egg: Whole	1 med.	50	235
White	1 med.	33	0
Yolk	1 med.	17	235
Fish, lean and medium fat, cooked	4 oz.	113	79
very fat, cooked	4 oz.	113	90
Gefilte Fish	3 oz.	85	54
Heart, cooked	3 oz.	85	119
Ham, cooked, trimmed	4 oz.	113	102
cooked, untrimmed	4 oz.	113	113
Ice Cream	1 scoop	71	43
Ice Milk	1 scoop	71	4
Kidney, cooked, no fat added	3 oz.	85	298
Lamb, cooked, trimmed	4 oz.	113	102
cooked, untrimmed	4 oz.	113	113
Lard and other animal fat	1 tbsp.	14	14-17
Liver, cooked, no fat added	3 oz.	85	213
Margarine, all vegetable fat	1 pat	7	0
Mayonnaise and mayonnaise-type salad dressing	1 tbsp.	14	8
Milk: Fluid, whole	1 cup	244	27
Fluid, skim	1 cup	246	0
Pork, cooked, trimmed	4 oz.	113	102
cooked, untrimmed	4 oz.	113	113
Shellfish: Clams, Crab, Lobster, Mussels, Shrimp, cooked	4 oz.	113	170
Sweetbreads, cooked	3 oz.	85	249
Tongue, cooked fresh	3 oz.	85	119
cooked smoked	3 oz.	85	179
Veal, cooked, trimmed	4 oz.	113	102
cooked, untrimmed	4 oz.	113	113

Note: Cholesterol is not present in foods of plant origin such as fruits, vegetables, cereal grains, legumes, nuts or oils.

APPENDIX D

OBESITY STANDARDS FOR CAUCASIAN AMERICANS[1]

(minimum triceps skinfold thickness in millimeters indicating obesity)[2]

Age (years)	Skinfold measurements Males	Skinfold measurements Females
5	12	14
6	12	15
7	13	16
8	14	17
9	15	18
10	16	20
11	17	21
12	18	22
13	18	23
14	17	23
15	16	24
16	15	25
17	14	26
18	15	27
19	15	27
20	16	28
21	17	28
22	18	28
23	18	28
24	19	28
25	20	29
26	20	29
27	21	29
28	22	29
29	23	29
30-50	23	30

[1] Adapted from Seltzer, C. C., and Mayer, J. A simple criterion of obesity. *Postgrad Med.* 38 : A 101-107, 1965.

[2] Figures represent the logarithmic means of the frequency distributions plus one standard deviation.

TABLE OF DESIRABLE WEIGHTS FOR MEN AND WOMEN AGED 25 AND OVER

(in pounds according to height and frame, in indoor clothing)

MEN

Height Feet	Height Inches	Small Frame	Medium Frame	Large Frame
5	2	112-120	118-129	126-141
5	3	115-123	121-133	129-144
5	4	118-126	124-136	132-148
5	5	121-129	127-139	135-152
5	6	124-133	130-143	138-156
5	7	128-137	134-147	142-161
5	8	132-141	138-152	147-166
5	9	136-145	142-156	151-170
5	10	140-150	146-160	155-174
5	11	144-154	150-165	159-179
6	0	148-158	154-170	164-184
6	1	152-162	158-175	168-189
6	2	156-167	162-180	173-194
6	3	160-171	167-185	178-199
6	4	164-175	172-190	182-204

WOMEN

Height Feet	Height Inches	Small Frame	Medium Frame	Large Frame
4	10	92- 98	96-107	104-119
4	11	94-101	98-110	106-122
5	0	96-104	101-113	109-125
5	1	99-107	104-116	112-128
5	2	102-110	107-119	115-131
5	3	105-113	110-122	118-134
5	4	108-116	113-126	121-138
5	5	111-119	116-130	125-142
5	6	114-123	120-135	129-146
5	7	118-127	124-139	133-150
5	8	122-131	128-143	137-154
5	9	126-135	132-147	141-158
5	10	130-140	136-151	145-163
5	11	134-144	140-155	149-168
6	0	138-148	144-159	153-173

Desirable weight tables are based on the concept that once growth in height has ceased there is no biological need to gain weight and that the best health prognosis (as reflected by mortality and morbidity data) is found in individuals of average or less than average weight in their early 20's. Desirable Weight Tables are designed to be applied to individuals aged 25 and over; measurements are with indoor clothing and shoes.

The Chart is adapted from insurance tables which are derived from the 1959 Build and Blood Pressure Study, Society of Actuaries. Three frame sizes are used, with a range of weights for each rather than a single weight. Unfortunately, no indication is given as to how to estimate frame size.

Acknowledgements

David B. Coursin, M.D.
Lancaster, Pennsylvania and
J.A.M.A. 154:406, 1954
Figures 35a, 35b

John H. Crandon, M.D.
Boston, Massachusetts
Figures 42a, 42b, 42c

William J. Darby, M.D.
Nashville, Tennessee
Figure 38

M. Edward Davis, M.D.
University of Chicago
Printzker School of Medicine
Chicago, Illinois
Figure 47

Thomas R. Dawber, M.D.
Boston, Massachusetts and
Ann. N.Y. Acad. Sci. 107:539, 1963
Chart 1a

James M. Dunning, D.D.S.
Boston, Massachusetts and
Harvard University Press
Chart 8

Bernard S. Epstein, M.D.
Long Island Jewish Hospital
New Hyde Park, New York
Figures 14, 18a, 18b, 18c, 45

Stanley N. Gershoff, Ph.D.
School of Public Health,
Department of Nutrition
Harvard University
Boston, Massachusetts
Figures 34, 4c

Sam Granek, Ph.D.
Rockefeller University
New York, New York
Figure 22

M. K. Horwitt, Ph.D.
St. Louis University
School of Medicine
St. Louis, Missouri and
Arch. Int. Med. 87:682, 1951
Figures 28, 29

Normal Jolliffe, M.D. and
The Upjohn Company
Figures 12a, 12b

Michael C. Latham, M.D.
Graduate School of Nutrition,
Cornell University
Ithaca, New York
*Figures 1, 3a, 3b, 4, 6, 11
19, 20, 21, 24, 31*

Richard H. Lyons, M.D.
State University of New York
Upstate Medical Center
Syracuse, New York
Figure 33

F. J. Margolis, M.D. *et al.*
Wayne State University,
College of Medicine
Kalamazoo, Michigan
Charts 2, 3, 4, 5

Karl E. Mason, Ph.D.
Bethesda, Maryland
Figures 46a, 46b

Rustin McIntosh, M.D.
Tyringham, Massachusetts
Figure 41

D. S. McLaren, M.D.
American University
of Beirut, Lebanon
and Bull. of World Health Org.
34:357, 1966
Figures 8, 10

Metropolitan Life Insurance Company
New York, New York
Appendix D

C. V. Moore, M.D.
St. Louis, Missouri
Figures 39a, 39b

National Health Education Committee, Inc.
New York, New York and
Department of Health,
Education and Welfare,
National Center for Health Statistics
Washington, D.C.
Chart 1b

Hildery A. Nelson, M.D.
Jamestown, New York
Figures 15, 16a, 16b

Rosa Lee Nemir, M.D.
New York University,
School of Medicine
New York, New York
Figure 43

Anthony J. Radford
Papua Medical College
Kainantuehd,
Territory of Papua
and New Guinea
Figure 4a

Blair C. Rich, D.D.S., F.I.C.D.
Rexburg, Idaho
*Figures 2a, 2b, 23
Charts 6, 7*

Carl C. Seltzer, Ph.D.
Department of Nutrition,
Harvard, University
Boston, Massachusetts
Appendix D

Karl Singer, M.D.
Chicago, Illinois
Figures 37a, 37b

Charley Smith, M.D.
University of Colorado
Medical Center
Denver, Colorado
Figure 40

Tom Spies, M.D. and
The Upjohn Company
Figures 25a, 25b, 25c, 27a, 27b, 32a, 32b

John C. Stalker, Director
Office of School Lunch Programs
and Nutrition Education
Department of Education,
Commonwealth of Massachusetts
Boston, Massachusetts
Figure 4d

Fredrick J. Stare, M.D.
School of Public Health,
Department of Nutrition
Harvard University
Boston, Massachusetts
Figures 4b, 5, 9

The Upjohn Company
Kalamazoo, Michigan
*Figures 7, 12a, 12b, 13a, 13b,
17a, 17b, 17c, 25a, 25b, 25c,
26a, 26b, 26c, 27a, 27b, 30,
32a, 32b, 36a, 36b, 48a, 48b, 48c*